Praise for The Pregnant Pause of Grief

"Personally, I found this book to be a source of inspiration for overcoming fear and uncertainty. This honest and heart rendering account of painful loss and precious memories is an amazing testimony of God's grace and the strength *He* provides in the midst of adversity. I thoroughly enjoyed the good humor and insightful dialogue and I highly recommend The Pregnant Pause of Grief for any of life's challenging situations."

~Lori Ciccanti, author of *From My Heart To Yours*
(Inspirational messages from the Wives of Ministers)
Ocean View, DE, USA

"This writing is not just another book on Grief, although that topic is the focus. It could lead one through any of life's struggles. *The Pregnant Pause of Grief: the First Trimester of Widowhood* describes biblical principles and teachings about how to not only "survive", but to grow out the other side as a stronger person. Brenda Wood's personal and transparent style of writing moves one from the initial feeling of overpowering loss to specific grounding concepts, anchoring the reader to move on realistically. Imagine an author who can incorporate occasional bits of personal humour, tucked into the volume of normal healthy tears. As a Christian Psychotherapist, I gladly recommend this book for persons who are working through the pain of grief."

~Suzanne Cantor Cameron, MSW, RSW, Psychotherapist
Toronto, ON, Canada

"I loved this book! It is a great read for anyone coming to grips with the loss of a spouse. The interspersing of scripture and personal anecdotes, make it an easy read. It will tug at your heart as you place your hand on the page and say, "I felt that too!" I would recommend this book to all new widows or widowers as they start this journey with God."

~Gina Kelly Ellis, Writer, Columnist for *Making a Difference*
Texas, USA

"Immediately following the passing of my wife I had the opportunity to read a draft of Brenda's book. Her writings really minister to me as I go through the grieving process and will continue to do so."

~Allan Smith, Worship leader and writer
Toronto, ON, Canada

I finished reading your manuscript today. I know it will help others who have lost loved ones. It helped me realize that I need to turn all of my fears over to God--daily. Thank you for that.

Tracy Campbell
www.tracycampbellwriter.wordpress.com

The First Trimester of Widowhood

The PREGNANT PAUSE of *Grief*

Brenda J. Wood

THE PREGNANT PAUSE OF GRIEF
Copyright © 2013 by Brenda J. Wood

All rights reserved. Neither this publication nor any part of this publication may be reproduced or transmitted in any form or by any means, electronic or mechanical, including photocopying, recording or any information storage and retrieval system, without permission in writing from the author.

All Scripture quotations, unless otherwise specified, are taken from the Amplified Bible, Copyright © 1954, 1958, 1962, 1964, 1965, 1987 by The Lockman Foundation. Used by permission. • Scripture quotations marked (MSG) are taken from The Message. Copyright © 1993, 1994, 1995, 1996, 2000, 2001, 2002. Used by permission of NavPress Publishing Group. • Scripture quotations marked (KJV) are taken from the King James Version of the Bible. • Scripture quotations marked (NKJV) or "New King James Version" are taken from the New King James Version / Thomas nelson Publishers, Nashville: Thomas Nelson Publishers, Copyright ©1982. Used by permission. All rights reserved. • Scripture taken from the New Century Version®. Copyright © 2005 by Thomas Nelson, Inc. Used by permission. All rights reserved. • Scripture quotations marked (NASB) are taken from the NEW AMERICAN STANDARD BIBLE®, Copyright © 1960, 1962, 1963, 1968, 1971, 1972, 1973, 1975, 1977, 1995 by The Lockman Foundation. Used by permission. • Scripture quotations marked (NLT) are taken from the Holy Bible, New Living Translation, copyright © 1996, 2004, 2007 by Tyndale House Foundation. Used by permission of Tyndale House Publishers, Inc., Carol Stream, Illinois 60188. All rights reserved. • Scripture quotations marked (NIV) are taken from the HOLY BIBLE, NEW INTERNATIONAL VERSION®. NIV®. Copyright© 1973, 1978, 1984 by International Bible Society. Used by permission of Zondervan. All rights reserved. • Scripture quotations marked (TLB) or "The Living Bible" are taken from the Living Bible / Kenneth N. Taylor. Wheaton: Tyndale house, 1997, c1971 by Tyndale House Publishers, Inc. Used by permission. All rights reserved.

Printed in Canada

ISBN: 978-1-77069-790-4

Word Alive Press
131 Cordite Road, Winnipeg, MB R3W 1S1
www.wordalivepress.ca

Cataloguing in Publication information available from Library and Archives Canada

As my husband Ron would say,
"Thank you muchly" for sharing our journey. May this
book help you, in some small way, toward your own healing.

What Is Our Script?

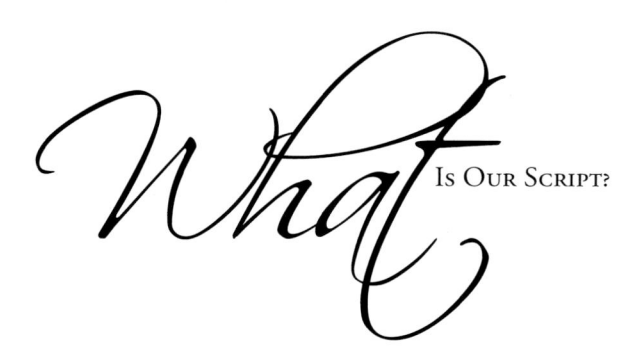

1

BY THE END OF THIS MONTH, I EXPECT TO KNOW MY OWN NAME. My friend didn't know hers for three months. Just past two now, I realize I, too, hardly know my own name. Some days, thick fog separates me from who I am or where I am. Pregnant with grief, hormones out of whack, and tears pouring forth for no reason, I encourage this new life within me. I struggle to believe it will come to full term and separate itself from me.

Perhaps you too find yourself struggling in your current life situation. You feel alone as you creep through this thing. Maybe, like me, you wonder if God still cares. I desperately search for the truth. I invite you to join me as we find out together.

My life situation is that I've become this new creature called "Widow." Ron died about two months ago. If you include our dating years, we spent fifty years as a couple. Together we trusted in this Bible verse: "*For I know the thoughts and plans that I have for you, says the Lord, thoughts and plans for welfare and peace and not for evil, to give you hope in your final outcome*" (Jeremiah 29:11).

I'm reading plans now that I do not care for at all. How can Ron's death give me hope and a future? How can this plan prosper and not harm me? Nothing about Ron's passing seems good. On the other hand, God has a reputation for being good. Maybe that's the difference.

I recently heard a TV message about this being our best life. The speaker insisted that we choose happiness every day. "Let's see you lose your spouse and still say those same words and mean them!" I shouted.

That frightened me. Where did those thoughts come from? I believed in God's best for me, didn't I? Still, how could anyone (especially me!) lose their beloved other half and continue to choose happiness?

That event led me on this path of self-discovery. A crisis calls us to evaluate what we believe about God and why we believe it. Do we really trust God the way we say we do? Do we really believe that His plans are better than ours? Don't we have to find out?

God says He loves us and insists His plans are the best. All He asks is that we trust Him and willingly follow His path. Is any of that even possible as we journey through heartbreaking grief?

One day at the doctor's office a young mom and her four-year-old twins kept us all in smiles. We needed a laugh because my darling husband, Ron, was suffering through the last stages of cancer. Hoping for a little peace and quiet, Mom picked a children's book off the shelf, arranged the little ones on either side, and began to read.

The girls did not like Mom's book one bit. It was one of those learn-your-alphabet things. They had no interest in A-B-Cs. They'd picked out happy cartoon-type books.

They begged and whined for Mom to discard her plan and use their particular picture books. The disappointed twins made a lot of noise, but Mom paid no attention. She calmly continued to read.

Eventually both girls set their books aside and listened to Mom's soft, gentle reading voice. The book she shared could prepare them for their life's journey. Her book could make a difference in the pathways they walked, the jobs they'd hold, and the income they'd earn. Mom gave them what they needed instead of what they wanted.

Can it be that God wants to teach us, but we don't care to learn? If we did, would we go the extra mile, build peace into our hearts, and enjoy wisdom in our souls? Does wisdom mean coming alongside God while He steadfastly points out new paths? Or does it mean acting like four-year-olds, demanding our own way? Surely that slows down the process of change and learning.

WHEN THE ANSWERS AREN'T
Lord, when our answers aren't there,
We question Your motives.
When our answers don't come,
We beg for relief.
When Your answers look different,
We cry out, "Not right!"
But all of that time
You're reading our story.
You whisper, "Just trust Me.
I've planned for your best.

>   I know where we're going.
>   Just hang on and rest."

I keep finding messages like Psalm 40:1-2:
"I waited patiently and expectantly for the Lord; and He inclined to me and heard my cry. He drew me up out of a horrible pit [a pit of tumult and of destruction], out of the miry clay (froth and slime), and set my feet upon a rock, steadying my steps and establishing my goings."

And Habakkuk 3:17–19:
Though the fig tree does not blossom and there is no fruit on the vines, [though] the product of the olive fails and the fields yield no food, though the flock is cut off from the fold and there are no cattle in the stalls, Yet I will rejoice in the Lord; I will exult in the [victorious] God of my salvation! The Lord God is my Strength, my personal bravery, and my invincible army; He makes my feet like hinds' feet and will make me to walk [not to stand still in terror, but to walk] and make [spiritual] progress upon my high places [of trouble, suffering, or responsibility]!

I've trusted God and His promises for years. Will they hold true in widowhood? I don't know yet.

I'm reading my journal scribbles again, reminding myself of times when God proved His faithfulness. Will I come to the same conclusions as I did then? Will I continue to trust Him, even in this most terrible time of my life? God never failed me before. Is it likely He will now?

I invite you to travel your painful journey with me. Let's remember how God met us in our worst places and brought good from each one.

In the past I learned that when the way is rough, our faith has a chance to grow. Is this still true? Is God still who He says He is? If He is, then through these new experiences we'll become the biggest mountain of faith you ever saw. Maybe mine is hiding in my twenty extra pounds! In that case, I'd better not lose it!

Are We Willing to Play the Waiting Game?

2

Everyone says, "Don't move a muscle yet. Wait at least a year before making big changes, selling the house, or changing investments."

Wait. Wait. Wait! That's easy to do. I hardly move a muscle. Inertia coats my body. All I do is weep. I get so sick of crying, of being surprised by tears. They surface when I least expect it. A whiff of Old Spice cologne, a John Deere symbol, or some other little thing reminds me of Ron, and I am a puddle.

I used to love grocery shopping because I'd hunt out low-fat or sugar-free items to make Ron's diabetic diet enjoyable. Now, shelves of low-cal products reduce me to tears. Shopping turns into aimless wandering. I meander up one store aisle, then down another.

For the first time ever, I look for something only for me. I buy one or two apples instead of a bag, two bananas rather than a bunch. Ron ate a sliced banana on his cereal every morning. He loved them over-ripe and practically oozing with juice. Ripe bananas give me migraines, and cereal hardly ever crosses my lips. The freezer already holds nine excessively brown bananas. Banana bread, you ask? Who will eat it?

My guy loved hamburger in any form. I eventually persuaded him away from the raw version. However, he never backed down from it cooked—that is, until the last few weeks of his life. Somehow his taste buds changed, and he even refused his favourite Wendy's burger (number 2). The family nicknamed that double patty "The Afi Burger." (*Afi* is Icelandic for Grandpa.) I wonder if that fast food chain kept it on the menu because they couldn't afford to take it off. Ron's donations kept them in business.

Note to self: Since Ron passed, the only foods I replace with regularity are coffee, peanut butter, and bread. Hmm. I need to branch out a bit. I do eat other things, but on a bad day those snacks become my meal.

Oh, note to others: Be careful what you tell your kids about your lifestyle. My life BR (before Ron passed) was one thing, and my life now, AR (after Ron), is quite another. AR includes rambling thought. Be patient. Just stay with me. Eventually, I'll get to the point.

Supposedly your concentration is a little off too. Stop wondering about your sanity. People who've lived through difficulties like ours insist we should not worry about this. Hopefully, the memory problems will eventually pass.

It must be a version of "baby brain." Some pregnant women apparently suffer from short-term memory loss, but that allows them to focus on their unborn children. Some believe this

THE PREGNANT PAUSE OF GRIEF

makes them better moms. If we follow that line of thinking, grief is making us into better widows or widowers. Meanwhile, let us meander at will.

One day AR, I made potato salad for a family gathering. The best potato salad gets made a day early, so the flavours meld. Well, I made this huge potato salad on Friday for the party on Saturday. When it came time for Friday lunch, the fridge held nothing but potato salad.

Potato salad makes the best sandwich filling. It's so yummy you can eat it for several meals in a row. However, if you tell your family things like this, they question you constantly about what, if anything, goes into your mouth. They query whether or not you are cooking for yourself. And you want to tell them what you think about their inquisitiveness. Don't. They fear losing you too. Remind yourself that they ask because they care.

Experts insist that we express our pain. Some people find this quite boring. "I've moved on," they say. "Why haven't you? Get over it. What's done is done."

Peter wept tears of guilt when he disowned Jesus three times. (See Luke 22:62.) Maybe somebody told him the same thing. "Get over it. What's done is done." And just maybe he couldn't see that happening anywhere in the near future. Still, it did, and he did, and God did. So maybe there is hope for the rest of us.

If you find someone who listens when you need to talk, holds your hand when you cry, and keeps his or her mouth shut (all at the same time), keep that diamond-studded personality in your life. Such gems are few and rare.

Lots of people go through hard times. Their advice is worth listening to. The opinions of those who have not suffered as you have may be well-meant but are pretty much worthless.

My immediate family listens, but they suffer their own pain. Often I hold back on mine to support them. After all, they've lost their much-loved Dad and their Afi, their precious Grandpa.

Healing happens as emotions squish out of us one way or another. That might mean loud weeping or heavy sighing, quiet reminiscing or snuggling in bed with blankets over our head for a day. Emotions must be dealt with. Release them in a safe place. You'll be able to figure out where that is soon enough. One Sunday afternoon, I wrapped myself in both Ron's housecoat and his leather jacket and just cried my eyes out.

Not everyone cries physical tears. Some people only cry on the inside. Grief experts say, "Do what is right for you." Tears apparently have hormones and actually help heal us as we shed them. Man, oh man! I sure must be healing a bunch.

I mourn my way through life; is there an end of it? I mean, after all, the Bible says, "*It came to pass*" (Genesis 4:3, KJV). It never says it came to stay. Perhaps I believe God more than I can recognize right now.

God says that "*Two are better than one, because they have a good [more satisfying] reward for their labor; For if they fall, the one will lift up his fellow. But woe to him who is alone when he falls and has not another to lift him up!*" (Ecclesiastes 4:9–10).

When calls, cards and letters stop coming, we are the ones who must pick up the phone, visit, or call the church office or counsellor. That's just the way it is. Others simply don't realize how thick the fog is or how overpowering the inertia.

A Fall Is More Than a Season

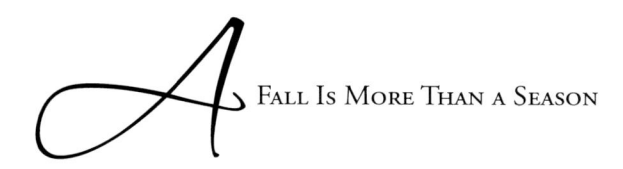

3

Last week, I had a nasty fall. It was my first time back out on the speaking circuit since Ron "passed."

I thoroughly dislike the word *died*. It's so final. I guess it is meant to be. After all, it *is* final, isn't it? It's the final of so many things for me. It's the final of our conjoined hearts. It ends our physical relationship and our earthly fellowship. As we delve deeper into pain, we'll find it is the end of so much more.

Anyway, back to that fall. An extra long staircase was the only way in or out of that place. Now, I might be wrong on that. I don't notice as much as I used to "BR." Maybe there was an elevator. If so, it totally escaped my notice. Anyway, I'd finished my speech, said all my goodbyes, and headed up those stairs carrying my briefcase full of books. Even at the bottom step, I thought, *There are so many stairs, and I am so tired.* Did I neglect to mention the weariness that accompanies this package? Sorry.

Just as my foot touched the top step, I thought, *I am going to fall.* And I did. Backwards down all those stairs.

The books only went halfway. Go figure. Me? I went all the way to the bottom. All the while I'm thinking, *How many more stairs can there be?* And, *Oh, that hurt! I'll need an x-ray of my cheekbone.*

I landed on my bottom, glasses still on but bent grotesquely out of shape, brain still sensible, body functioning, and mouth spitting bits of tooth. People came running to see what the "big thumping sounds" were. Note to Brenda: Lose that extra twenty pounds!

"Well," I said, jokingly, "now when I watch all those cowboy movies, I'll know how they fell out of those buildings." Nobody laughed. I'm sure they thought me quite insensible from the fall.

"Call nine-one-one," cried one.

"Get a chair," cried another.

"Get her off the floor," ordered someone else.

Actually, I felt quite comfortable on the floor and did not care to move one inch over, let alone up.

"I'll get a glass of water," said one.

All the while, my tummy rumbled the thought *Swallow nothing for fear of something coming back up!*

Everyone has a "fix" in life. Generally, their fix for you is what they would like under the same circumstances. It's all they can do, and they want to do something. It's hardly ever what you want or need.

Thankfully, no one called 911. Perhaps their cellphones were out of commission. I was relieved. I wanted to get over my own pain in my own way and at my own non-breakneck speed. After all, I wasn't broken, only bent.

THE PREGNANT PAUSE OF GRIEF

No matter. They hauled me up on that chair. This made others more comfortable. Me? Not so much.

I swallowed small sips of water, twice, but I sure didn't want them. I've always had trouble saying no to well-meaning people and, yes, even to those who do not have my well-being at heart. We'll talk more about that later.

Anyway, those dear ladies enjoyed doing what they wanted to do to make me feel more comfortable. I admit I was a little dazed. You try hanging upside down and sideway for several seconds and see how you feel. Think of your last amusement ride and how nauseating that was. Whew! So that was me.

"Let us drive you home."

I considered the trouble this would cause. I really wanted to be alone to evaluate what happened anyway.

"No, thanks. I will be fine. I can drive myself."

"Are you dizzy?"

"No, I am not nor was I ever dizzy." I did not say this aloud for fear of hurting their feelings.

"What happened? Did you trip?"

"No, I don't think so…I just had the thought that I was going to fall."

Note to self: Check out *Battlefield of the Mind* by Joyce Meyer (New York: Time Warner, 2004). How much power did my thought create towards my fall? What if I'd thought "I'm almost at the top; I can make it"?

The gals continued to bombard me with questions, while I just craved peace and quiet.

"How far did you get up the stairs before you fell?"

"I had my foot on that top step. Second from the bottom would have made a more pleasant landing." Again, no one laughed. Had I lost my sense of humour in the downward flight?

"What can we do for you?"

"Nothing, thanks. Please help me up those stairs. Could someone carry my books please?"

I answered all their questions because that's what they needed. One question finished me off.

"Do you want us to call your husband?"

With that, my true feelings escaped.

I whispered the words I hate to hear. "He died two months ago."

That dear darling gal hugged me and said nothing. I don't think she told the others, because no one rushed up to console me. What a relief! My feelings escaped into the air, but a safe listener held on to them for me. Quite frankly, I had no inclination to spend any more words on the subject.

We are hedged in (pressed) on every side [troubled and oppressed in every way], but not cramped or crushed; we suffer embarrassments and are perplexed and unable to find a way out, but not driven to despair; We are pursued (persecuted and hard driven), but not deserted [to stand alone]; we are struck down to the ground, but never struck out and destroyed (2 Corinthians 4:8–9).

All the while, I'd been gently massaged my glasses into some sort of order so that the left arm no longer pointed north and the lenses east. If the crowd had ever seen those frames in such disarray, I'd never have been permitted out on my own.

Finally, I tried to stand alone. Everyone hovered. They were obviously concerned.

"I can drive myself home," I declare firmly.

"Really?" they asked. "Are you sure?"

Yes, I am sure. Convinced that my body is intact, I gently test the waters of standing. Funny, I only hurt beside my left eye, where rugburn discolours my skin to a scarlet hue.

"You're not bleeding," someone says.

I think, *At least on the outside I'm not bleeding. My heart is broken and bleeding on the inside, but no one can fix that.* Pain resulting from this fall cannot begin to touch the oozing wound resonating in my heart.

Someone helped me up the stairs. Another carried books. That meant I hadn't missed the elevator, right? If there was one, surely they'd have offered it to a gamely waddling, weak-kneed stranger who couldn't make the stairs the first time when she wasn't gamely waddling and weak-kneed!

I asked for an easier way home, and the crowd offered helpful suggestions. I smiled, nodded, and let the words slide over and out, like an old-fashioned CB radio call. God and I would find our way.

I drove in the direction I hoped might be the highway. I finally spotted the sign after a few blocks, but I couldn't swerve fast enough into the correct lane. So up and around a few times I went. Turning in driveways here and there, turning and returning, until finally that quiet road and I met as one.

Today, I avoided briskly moving traffic-jammed freeways. I headed north along sultry side streets with multiple stop signs, toward the safe harbour of my little home. I'm glad I paid some attention BR when Ron used to map out my journeys.

Dare to Evaluate Life Experiences Through More Than the Physical

4

WITH MY ATTENTION FIRMLY ON THE ROAD—WELL, AS MUCH attention as a wonky person is able to give—my only thought was to get my glasses straightened. I reasoned that if only I could see properly, all would be well.

What a lie! I doubt anything will feel "well" to me ever again. Personal lies are believable when you're desperate.

"God, I was out speaking for You. Where were You? What am I supposed to learn from this experience?"

Funny, I never asked God that when Ron died. I wonder why. Didn't I want to learn anything? Was I in shock or afraid of the answers? I don't know, so I concentrated on that fall.

Yes, I was overtired. I said "Yes" when I should have said "No." Not to the Bible studies I teach or to my little part-time job. Not to family time, either, but to all the other events that left me consoling others when I couldn't yet even find comfort myself.

Ron and I always protected each other.

"Brenda is too busy to go there right now."

"Ron is not feeling well enough to take that on. Sorry."

We buffered each other, but now my buffer is gone, so I repeatedly take on obligations that leave me no time to lock the door, rest, and search for recovery from this life trauma.

Still, it was the first time I'd spoken professionally since Ron died. I suspect that certain other world forces found that unappealing. Did the way I fell mirror my current life? Thoughts like "How many more stairs can there be?" translated easily into "How much longer does this feeling of loss last?" I already know the answer to that question, and you do too. Maybe it's forever.

Glasses all cockeyed? Perhaps I wasn't seeing my world quite as clearly as I should have, but the glasses stayed on. Perhaps only my vision needed adjustments. Where was God? Had He suffered with me while I tumbled?

He did prevent broken bones, but He didn't prevent the fall, or any of the multiple bruises that appeared over the next week. He gave me strength for the journey home. He kept an eye clinic open so a total stranger could repair my glasses and restore my vision. I decided that my spiritual vision needed to trust God more, while trusting myself less. That seemed the most important deduction of all.

I thought about the prayer of Jabez.

"Jabez cried to the God of Israel, saying, Oh, that You would bless me and enlarge my border, and that Your hand might be with me, and You would keep me from evil so it might not hurt me! And God granted his request" (1 Chronicles 4:10).

God continues to enlarge my borders. Three writing awards came my way in the last month. I've been invited to speak at several new venues. I'm writing 50,000 words this month. I'm on a roll, but I roll forward without my right arm. I've never had to do that before.

Fifty years is a long time. How can a gal get over a loss like that in less time than it takes to brush her teeth?

A friend wrote these soothing words of consolation:

"I just wanted to say I feel your sorrow. It's normal, and will become a familiar attendee at the table with you; even when you get used to it, it bubbles up in the most unexpected places. What is now normal is transient and will in time settle down to a new normality. When God says that the two become one flesh, He means it. You're suffering with—pardon the pun—a phantom limb. Your brain says Ron should be there, but he is not. The Grace of God overwhelms the temporary sorrow for those who suffer presently."

That states it exactly, but I ask myself which limb is missing—my extra ear, my right arm, or the feet that walked beside me? Perhaps it's the voice that whistled music to my ears or the smile that cascaded twinges of love into my heart. No, it must be that twinkling eye, the wink that said "I love you, Princess."

I ask you, which limb? Not one, but *all* of them. Every part of Ron is gone except the bits I remember, and they seem to be dwindling.

So now I'm off on a bunny trail, investigating phantom limbs. A phantom limb is the sensation that amputated or missing limbs, even an organ like the appendix, remains attached to the body and moves appropriately with other body parts. Phantom sensations may even occur after the removal of a breast, a tooth, or an eye. Sixty to eighty percent of amputees experience these painful phantom sensations, so why wouldn't it occur after other losses, like death?

The missing limb may feel cramped into distorted and painful positions. Of course! I understand now why every movement wrenches and rips asunder everything I know and love.

Apparently phantom limb pain worsens in times of stress, anxiety, and weather changes. That's easy to figure. Stress makes us into blithering idiots anyway. Just the other day, when I thought about winterizing the house and keeping up with the snow, I burst into tears, totally overwhelmed. Thankfully, after I made just one reaching-out phone call, the family responded within the hour. Openings got covered, air conditioner sealed, and snow removal organized.

And that weather? Who doesn't dummy down into morose feelings on a rainy Saturday? Who doesn't wish for a little sunshine? Did God make gloomy weather so we would reach out for His Son just from the sheer missing of Him?

Phantom limb pain is usually intermittent. Frequency and intensity may decline over time. I sure hope so. One gal told me that every day gets a little brighter; otherwise, how could we go on living? Such a high level of nervous anxiety and stressful struggle would be impossible to put up with forever. Surely that's why God comforts as He does. Surely after we live through the first Thanksgiving, birthday and Christmas in that "new" normal, surely then the phantom grief must subside a bit.

Some people's phantom limbs feel and behave as though they are still attached. For the griever that would be the same as making decisions based only on what the dearly departed would do. I want to do that.

THE PREGNANT PAUSE OF GRIEF

Like that winterizing thing. Ron always put plastic all around the porch, both front and back. The family and I ended up covering the lawn chairs and the rest with plastic and leaving the walls as is. That is definitely not a Ron-do. But for us this year, in our grieving state, it's all we can manage. "Used to" cannot be our measuring stick. What would God do? That is the better gauge.

Some people's phantom limbs take on a life of their own, disobeying the owner's commands. I bet this would happen if we did not deal wisely with our troubles. What if we stopped our lives right where they were? What if we left everything in its place? What if we didn't clear out our beloved's clothes?

I know of a woman who kept her husband's entire wardrobe after he was lost in the Second World War. She insisted he'd want his fine tailored suits and shirts when he came back. Years later, that clothing still haunted her every new home. She continued to cling to those rags; by then, they really were rags. They replaced previously cherished memories, as out-of-date as those 1930s suits.

The theory is that the brain keeps the memory of the limb's positions. We see that something is missing, but our brain remembers the limb as a functioning body part. Yes! I notice Ron is not in his Big Red Chair. (Note: I wrote the children's book *The Big Red Chair* to comfort our grandchildren after Ron died.) I see that he's not sitting beside me on the way to church. I shop alone. The double bed might as well be single. I put his pillow to my back at night, pretending that his body snuggles mine. The pots and pans hold food for one. I cherish memories of our picnic-style meals on the front porch, and I long for his all-embracing hugs.

A dear family friend, Margaret, once waxed poetic over those hugs:

21

BRENDA J. WOOD

A Ron Wood hug makes me feel better than
chocolate chip ice cream
or fresh-picked cherries
or presents under the tree
or strawberries in cream
or buttercups
or big pink balloons
or puppies
or stories with happy endings
or baby elephants
or diamonds
or jumping in puddles
or bluebells and primroses.
Better than bare feet in dewy grass
or favourite records
or letters from old friends
or gypsy caravans
or campfires and glow-worms.
Better than rainbows
or summer sunsets over the water
or the sound of the sea
or the birds' dawn chorus
or organ music.
Better than dancing
or feeling sand between one's toes
or lovely old houses
or walking in the rain
or hearing the choir on Christmas Eve
or smelling wood smoke on an autumn evening
or my stuffed dog…
Better than—well—just better. That's all.
I guess he had a good teacher.
She makes hugs special, too.
(Margaret Parrot, used by permission)

THE PREGNANT PAUSE OF GRIEF

My beloved hugger is gone, and with that, I've also lost my position as huggee. I forget, and sometimes I speak aloud my thoughts about a news event or turn on his favourite game show and pretend…but it is all pretend.

Maybe the beginning of healing is realizing that it's all pretend. After all, isn't that what Solomon said? *"I have seen all the works that are done under the sun, and behold, all is vanity, a striving after the wind and a feeding on wind"* (Ecclesiastes 1:14).

Perhaps someday, vision and memory will connect their dots and become one, like Ron and I became one over fifty years. If not, like the suit-holder, I'll be one of those stuck people, never recovering from grief but carrying it forever, allowing it to become my defining life moment. Even in my current state, I recognize how unhealthy that would be. Thanks, but no thanks.

Some phantom-pain experts suggest drugs to block amputees' memories so they won't remember the actual amputation. Others think that drugs could get us through our troubles. They insist that we don't have to "feel like this." Actually, I think we do. If we don't allow ourselves to feel awful now, how will we recognize when we're feeling better?

Other phantom-pain treatments include vibration therapy, acupuncture, hypnosis, and biofeedback, but apparently they don't help much. Pain is minimized by keeping busy and focusing one's attention on something else.

Yes! If we let our minds dwell on the past, the pain, and the loneliness, we get stuck there. But by moving ourselves into today and refusing to panic over either past or future, we do better. When God helps us "battle our minds" into their right places, surely we will begin to trust Him more. Won't we?

Note: The fall occurred because I took a stomach drug that tires you out, wears you down, and makes you weary…*Now* they tell me!

Meandering

Is Normal During Emotional Shock

5

Someone sends me a prayer: "May God's ever-present hope in times of trouble grant you His perfect peace and consolation today and set you in His family of love."

I suppose we can refuse to accept the "new normal." What if we can't trust our feelings? None of us appreciates overwhelming sorrow when we least expect it. We don't want to cry after innocuous comments like "How are you doing?" We don't want to take offence when others ask why we don't do this or that. We don't want to—but sometimes we do.

Doing? I'm not even being! I barely toddle to the coffee pot in the morning. For years, I set up the coffee pot the night before. If I ever forgot, I'd make it by the light of the fridge. That way Ron could get the extra sleep he so badly needed.

Now I make it with the lights on, because the old way, from when his darling head slept on the pillow next to mine, makes me cry. Tears may assault us but sometimes we do self-induce.

It's hard to type when you can't see the keys. My heart leaks badly today. All my words have a hodgepodge of weirdness about them. Laying out feelings for the world to see is a painful thing.

Just when I thought I couldn't do it, I got a note from a friend who unknowingly sent my favourite verse. *"I have strength for all things in Christ Who empowers me [I am ready for anything and equal to anything through Him Who infuses inner strength into me; I am self-sufficient in Christ's sufficiency]"* (Philippians 4:13).

She added that her recent weight loss and daily exercise changed her life. She used to walk her bike up high hills. Now she greets hills with wild abandon because almost no hill is beyond her trying.

Wait a minute! It's the "trying," isn't it? If we don't try, how will we know whether we can climb our particular hill? Are we actively pursuing heart healing or wallowing in the situation? Does getting over heartache mean leaving my darling Ron behind, forgetting who he was, what he looked like, and how much he loved me? Will memories stay firm or disappear in this overwhelming grief?

How many times do we look at something in our life and think this hill is too much for us to manage and go back to look for another, easier, route? Meanwhile the Father, arms outstretched, encourages us to move up that original hill toward Him. The Bible insists that we must keep our eyes on Jesus. What an example of hill climbing!

Looking away [from all that will distract] to Jesus, Who is the Leader and the Source of our faith [giving the first incentive for our belief] and is also its Finisher [bringing it to maturity and perfection]. He, for the joy [of obtaining the prize] that was set before Him, endured the cross, despising and ignoring the shame, and is now seated at the right hand of the throne of God (Hebrews 12:2).

I cry out, "Lord, this immensely giant, fearful issue looms ahead of us. We're holding on to You for dear life, because if we don't, we'll fall, collapse, or disintegrate. God, don't drop us."

Then I remember that

"He [God] Himself has said, I will not in any way fail you nor give you up nor leave you without support. [I will] not, [I will] not, [I will] not in any degree leave you helpless nor forsake nor let [you] down (relax My hold on you)! [Assuredly not!]" (Hebrews 13:5).

Whew! What a relief.

I'm an oldest child and a type A personality. I want to control everything. What if this overachiever rested, let feelings go, and trusted God instead? What if I allowed myself kindness, gentleness, and understanding? What if I treated myself as generously as I treat others?

I think about the publicity lines on my blog: "I believe Jesus is the answer to every question." If that's true, shouldn't I allow the God of all comfort to comfort me? Doesn't He promise that He is our comforter in our sorrow, when our hearts are faint within us? (From Jeremiah 8:18.)

Right now this motivational speaker can hardly dress in the morning, let alone motivate somebody else. I'm a recovering bulimic who's gained and lost thousands of pounds over the years. I understand the pain of being overweight and the agony of eating disorders, but am I still known for my common-sense wisdom, sense of humour, and quirky comments?

Water is hot at 211 degrees Fahrenheit, but at 212 degrees Fahrenheit it boils and gives off enough steam to power huge machinery. Is our personal circumstance hot enough to give off steam? Who motivates us that one extra degree? Dare we ask God to help us? Do we have to believe in order to ask?

They say if you can't stand the heat, get out of the kitchen. Life's "kitchen heat" fogs our decision-making. Is it hot enough to motivate us towards God?

I pray for wisdom and strength.

"Lord, we have so many questions and so few answers. Help us, God. Clarify our beliefs, even to ourselves. Tell us the truth. Help us love and believe You enough to live the way You say we can. Help us hang on through this morass of pain and grief. Don't let us fall spiritually like we do physically. Amen."

"*And let us not lose heart and grow weary and faint in acting nobly and doing right, for in due time and at the appointed season we shall reap, if we do not loosen and relax our courage and faint*" (Galatians 6:9). These verses also offer hope:

> *So I say to you, Ask and keep on asking and it shall be given you; seek and keep on seeking and you shall find; knock and keep on knocking and the door shall be opened to you. For everyone who asks and keeps on asking receives; and he who seeks and keeps on seeking finds; and to him who knocks and keeps on knocking, the door shall be opened* (Luke 11:9–10).

And this promise keeps us asking:

> *Also [Jesus] told them a parable to the effect that they ought always to pray and not to turn coward (faint, lose heart, and give up). He said, In a certain city there was a judge who neither reverenced and feared God nor respected or considered man. And there was a widow in*

THE PREGNANT PAUSE OF GRIEF

that city who kept coming to him and saying, Protect and defend and give me justice against my adversary. And for a time he would not; but later he said to himself, Though I have neither reverence or fear for God nor respect or consideration for man, Yet because this widow continues to bother me, I will defend and protect and avenge her, lest she give me intolerable annoyance and wear me out by her continual coming or at the last she come and rail on me or assault me or strangle me (Luke 18:1–5).

Silent noise and hot food cause tears. The house echoes of an empty life. Empty. In my BR life, I'd come home from work at dinnertime to find a pot of potatoes on the boil. Ron would have some kind of beef (his preference) on the barbecue. I'd push for vegetables and maybe a salad. We'd each eat a little of the other's choice, secretly grateful for our own. Now there remains nothing but deafening silence and me.

I work at eating the near-expiry-date stuff in the fridge. One night I decide to poach eggs. Ron didn't care for them. An egg meal meant I'd cook his scrambled eggs first, not because he demanded it but because that's how some of us love. We feed others and then ourselves. Our meals tend to be on the cool side. We don't notice; nor do we really care.

So I poached up those eggs. They were the best eggs I'd eaten in forty-eight years: hot, seasoned perfectly. And I cried, thinking how I'd willingly eat cold scrambled eggs forever, if only my Honey were here.

He's Never Too Early for the Christmas Tree

6

I'm late getting to the computer today because I decorated the little spruce tree on the north side of the yard. The park staff planted it about ten days before Ron died. We sat at the breakfast table and watched it going in.

"We'll decorate it for Christmas this year," I said. Ron didn't answer, but later I heard him tell his buddy, "Brenda says we'll decorate it this year."

That little tree stands bravely forth in its first holiday suit. Red bows, glittering baubles, and lights festoon it into merriness. I cried because it was supposed to be a "we" project.

A "we" project included putting plastic up around the back porch and wrapping the children's Christmas presents. We'd work on the special bacon and egg breakfast for the morning of December 25th. We fought the turkey into submission, stuffed it outrageously, and together we gasped as its legs fell off when we lifted it from the oven. A "we" project like our past forty-eight years. One half of "we" is me. Am *I* up to the job?

Yesterday I surprised myself with a good day, the first in a long time. Oh, there have been snatches of time here and there, an occasional laugh with friends, a smile of remembrance, but a whole day? Dare I hope for a future week or even a month absent from the overwhelming, crushing pain that crawls up from the depths of my soul and puddles my eyes? Medical people might deem this pathway from soul to eyes impossible, but haven't we all experienced it at one time or another?

If we force ourselves to think of other things, we might stave it off for a few minutes. But sometimes we want to think about our troubles, and if that makes rivers of makeup and lakes of tears in coffee cups, so be it. I've thought of Ron every day of my life since I was sixteen. I can't see myself stopping now. He's not that easy to forget.

I fill my personal abyss with everything but what it wants—Ronald M. Wood. Should I call someone, go for coffee, or find a dinner companion? None of these thoughts make me feel better. Not today, anyway.

I put on my housecoat…well, Ron's John Deere housecoat. I claimed it for my own shortly after he died, so that I could snuggle closer to him. My actions surely must sound pathetic, unless you too have experienced loss. That piece of fabric is never, ever, going to take the place of my darling. Quite the opposite, in fact, because it is like all the other paltry things I do to help myself cope. It's simply another reminder of his departure.

That first night, the funeral home folks, friends, and family left by 1 a.m. I wanted to be alone, talk to God, air my differences, weep, and rest and grieve alone. I took Ron's pillow from the hospital bed and put it back in bed with me where it belonged. Its John Deere pillowcase carried his scent. I buried my face in it, wanting to hold on and remember. I tucked his heart pillow, a relic from his heart surgery and recovery, against my chest and held on for dear life. I slept till 3 a.m., got up, and started laundry. Only our butternut-coloured sheets fit the hospital bed with its extra-deep mattress. I washed them first, wanting them back on our bed. They belonged, like my grief belonged, in the depths of the softness of our bedroom where we'd spent roughly one-third of our married life.

Do the math. We spend about eight hours out of every twenty-four in bed. No wonder that bed comforts me so. Now, two months later, I still sniff that pillowcase, pretending that some sweet scent of Ron remains. I wear the housecoat. The heart pillow still comforts me. I find ways to help myself cope because otherwise I travel backwards. I already did that when I fell. Never again.

You can quit a job, leave a family, or buy a house. Stop having children, eat chocolate, or do the laundry. Decorate, shop for shoes, or become a Christian. Everything else in life is a choice. Death is not.

Ron wouldn't have chosen it, and I surely didn't, yet here we are. Though I'm a wreck, I wouldn't want Ron to go through this. We talked about what we'd do if one of us died first. We firmly promised not to "lie down and die" because the other had gone.

"Oh, we will be strong," we insisted to each other.

We didn't have a clue what we were talking about. We didn't know we'd feel like a tree whose limbs struggle to hang on while a chainsaw gang saws and pulls away. Stuff wrenched from us makes our physical space all wrong, because there were two and now there is only one.

Think how we eat a doughnut. Our hands grab and yank. Bits that once belonged fall away; crust divides unevenly, and sprinkles scatter. The doughnut is still a doughnut though chewed, masticated, and devoured. A few misplaced sprinkles remain. Ron's death made me into a sprinkle.

Daily circumstances wrench Ron away. I'm expected to cancel his passport, his license, his pensions, and everything else. I fight still to get his name off the house insurance, or else for the rest of my life any claim cheque will say "Estate of Ronald M. Wood and Brenda Wood." I'd have to prove all over again that he died in order to cash the cheque. How crazy (and, I ask you, how painful) is that? Ron's will and death certificate mean nothing to the insurance company, even though everyone else (including the bank and the government) finds them adequate.

Government papers say he's no longer here; those same papers seriously deplete my income, leaving me financially unstable for months.

May I thank the fellow sufferers in my life? Experienced others understand that even a loaf of bread or a quart of milk might be unaffordable for the first few weeks. They learned the hard way that paying for a coffee at the local restaurant might break the budget. Secretly, quietly, one by one, they gave me donations out of their little bits.

"This is instead of flowers," they whispered.

We asked people to donate to our church and the local cancer clinic. Many did. But the experienced gave money gifts to me.

"Let me know if you don't have enough," they wrote.

"This bit will buy you milk and bread for a while."

And it did. My gifts from now on will not grant me a tax receipt but instead support a friend in possible need.

THE PREGNANT PAUSE OF GRIEF

Should I eat early tonight? Granny and Grandpa ate at four thirty, sharing a quiet meal before their boarders showed up at five. Boarders were their meal ticket when times were tough. When I stayed there, I slept on the couch because the other bedrooms were full of…you guessed it…boarders.

A "Cook" in more than maiden name, Gran shone at local fairs and bake sales. Her recipes read something like this: "Add one-half sugar-bowl of milk and one heaping thimbleful of baking soda." Unless I find both sugar bowl and thimble, I'm sunk.

To raise money for a new church pulpit Bible, Granny gave church members the opportunity to write their names on a quilt top. Then she charged them twenty-five cents for the privilege. She hand-embroidered the names, finished the quilt, and raffled it off. She made enough money to buy the Bible. In return, she got the old one and a thank-you letter from the church.

When I inherited it, I returned it, along with the letter. They'll restore it to its original beauty. I wish I knew where the quilt went. It likely wore out during its tour of duty, keeping the unheated warm.

Okay, so now I've calmed down a bit. Remembering Granny always does that to me. Dad said I'm exactly like her. He'd know, I guess. He lived a long time with both of us.

Granny, too, became a widow. Ron's mom, the same…They made a "new normal" life for themselves, and I know I will too. It's just that I don't feel too much like it today. So there!

I Can't Stand M.A.S.H.

7

Ron loved that show. Five o'clock sharp and our world stopped for those reruns. Truthfully, Ron watched alone. They were reruns, for goodness' sake. Been there, done that. I'd read, stir dinner, and even journal—anything to pass the time till six o'clock. That would mean dinner and the news and no M.A.S.H. Still, that show insidiously crept into my brain and implanted itself.

I loved hearing Ron laugh at those old predictable jokes. I enjoyed his occasional repeating of a line and secretly watched him when he wasn't looking. My heart gushed with love, and during the commercials I might say something like "I tell you that my heart bursts with loving you right this minute!" He'd grin, and I'd scramble across the room to give him a kiss.

Today I give M.A.S.H. another chance. Perhaps if I watch it, memories of Ron will burst joyfully forth. They burst all right. I recognize the next joke. I know the punch line. And I know Ron would laugh here, and say that, and I'd kiss him there.

M.A.S.H. and I part company. It's over for us. I flip to the cooking channel. No tears there unless they start chopping onions. At least there, the tears won't be mine.

I use Granny's trick, pulling Ron's John Deere housecoat over my clothes. If anyone comes to the door, a quick whip off of the green and yellow and I'm ready to go.

I search the TV for a movie. No, nothing I want to see. Music is out. Songs like "We Had It All," "American Pie," "Knock Three Times," and other favourites bombard me in quick succession. Ron and I danced through life. We knew every hit song because they'd accompanied us on dance floors somewhere.

An exceptional dancer, Ron made me look like I knew what I was doing. Not just modern hits either. Our polka, waltz, jive, and twist cleared the floor on several occasions and even won us a few prizes.

The last few years he didn't have so much energy as before, and, quite frankly, neither did I. His illnesses wore us both down, but we still danced. We called it Toe Dancing. Our song would come up, and one of us would call out, "Toe Dance!" We'd sit in our respective chairs, twisting and wriggling our toes to the music, all the while grinning at one another like Cheshire cats. Afterwards, I'd snuggle with him and get my kiss.

I know what you're thinking. You're thinking that I make Ron out to be perfect. You're thinking that I've closed my eyes to reality. You wonder about our big fights and battles. Truthfully, we seldom had any. Because our marriage held first

THE PREGNANT PAUSE OF GRIEF

place, anything that disrupted it took second. We learned to willingly forgive small things because of their very smallness.

We learned to love through God's eyes. We resolved that divorce would never be an option. We determined to help each other be all we could be in Christ. Ron believed in and lived the truth of Ephesians 5:28–31:

Even so husbands should love their wives as [being in a sense] their own bodies. He who loves his own wife loves himself. For no man ever hated his own flesh, but nourishes and carefully protects and cherishes it, as Christ does the church, because we are members (parts) of His body. For this reason a man shall leave his father and his mother and shall be joined to his wife, and the two shall become one flesh.

We loved each other more than we loved ourselves. That is the only way to make a marriage work. Relationships are not 50 percent from one person and 50 percent from the other. Each must contribute 100 percent. Sometimes one person gives 175 percent while the other only manages 25. Somehow that total has to make over 200 percent. I didn't always live that way until I heard the following comments from one aged widow.

Several of us married gals bemoaned the fact that our hubbies wouldn't do this or that. One woman couldn't even get her guy to take his (prepared by her) sandwich out of the fridge. He simply starved himself till she got home. We laughed and droned on.

One dear little widow turned from her stance at the kitchen sink, stared us all down, and spoke these life-changing words: "I'd give anything to be able to make lunch for my husband today."

Right then, my mind turned to life without my sweetie. That comment made a difference. I changed my words forever.

I decided to show Ron on a daily basis how much I loved and cherished him. I'm glad I did. Still, until he died, I couldn't sense how his death could sear such an indescribable parting in me.

I check the fridge. Tons of choices but none I care to eat. My Weight Watchers tracker tells me that I planned creamed cauliflower with fat-free milk and light cheese. Wow. What was I thinking? I cook the whole head of cauliflower. Maybe I'll want the rest tomorrow.

That is my din-din. Surprisingly, I find I am hungry. No cauliflower tomorrow. Anyway, it was one small lonely head. Already enough loneliness hanging around outside the crisper; no point in adding more.

I've always thought I could cheerfully be a vegetarian. This is a good time to find out. Granny didn't eat meat but piled vegetables up on her plate. Then she'd add a good sprinkle of pepper and a thick slice of her homemade bread. She made twelve loaves a week. Recall those hungry male boarders?

Once, after one of her heart attacks, I caught her eating a wallop of full-fat cottage cheese on top of a couple of poached eggs.

"Oh, that looks disgusting," I cried.

"You'd eat it too, if you had to." She grimaced.

"But together?" I cried. "Do you have to eat them together?"

That's the only time I ever saw Gran eat alone. She ate with folks so they'd eat well. She shared a cup of tea with boarders so they had a family-dining experience. She ate one-on-one with whoever came to visit, but she never seemed to eat alone. She must have after Gramps died. I'm ashamed to say, I never checked.

No one really checks here either, especially on the weekends. They enjoy family times, and if they give a thought to what

THE PREGNANT PAUSE OF GRIEF

a widow is doing, it is seldom with an eye to inviting one to dinner.

A friend redefines the word. She says *widow* in thought is dreaded, but in word *widow* stands for Wonderful Intelligent Daughter Of Wisdom. *Wonderful* is another word for "outstanding." One meaning of *intelligent* is "sensible or rational, the ability to think and understand things clearly and logically." Of course a daughter is a female child. And *wisdom* means "the ability to make sensible decisions and judgments based on personal knowledge and experience."

That leaves us with an outstanding, sensible, rational female child with the ability to make judgments based on personal knowledge and experience. That doesn't sound like a person with a foggy head.

In the biblical sense, Christ is our wisdom. "*In Him all the treasures of [divine] wisdom (comprehensive insight into the ways and purposes of God) and [all the riches of spiritual] knowledge and enlightenment are stored up and lie hidden*" (Colossians 2:3).

Let me repeat myself. What do we have here? We have an outstanding, sensible, rational female child with the ability to make judgments based on Christ's personal knowledge and experience. Now that is something to depend on. "*For skillful and godly Wisdom is better than rubies or pearls, and all the things that may be desired are not to be compared to it*" (Proverbs 8:11).

"*It is as sport to a [self-confident] fool to do wickedness, but to have skillful and godly Wisdom is pleasure and relaxation to a man of understanding*" (Proverbs 10:23). "*For the wisdom of this world is foolishness in God's sight*" (1 Corinthians 3:19, NIV). But is wisdom even possible in this world?

"*For the LORD gives wisdom; and from his mouth come knowledge and understanding*" (Proverbs 2:6, NIV). If He is the source of all wisdom, the next step must be to ask for it.

"If any of you lacks wisdom, you should ask God, who gives generously to all without finding fault, and it will be given to you" (James 1:5, NIV). Well then, let's get to the asking!

Oops! There is one condition.

"But when you ask, you must believe and not doubt, because the one who doubts is like a wave of the sea, blown and tossed by the wind. That person should not expect to receive anything from the Lord. Such a person is double-minded and unstable in all they do" (James 1:6–8, NIV).

Then let this be our prayer.

Let's keep asking God to give us a spirit of wisdom, so that we can get to know Him better! (From Ephesians 1:17–18.)

This widow cautiously dares to look beyond her present into a daring new future. I hope you'll join me.

Fear Is the Result of an Overly Active Imagination

8

"I'm telling you, 'Don't panic. I'm right here to help you'" (Isaiah 41:13).

When Ron broke his jaw in a work accident, he actually experienced God's handshake. (See "Ron's Story" in chapter 28.) After Ron moved to God Central, a friend pointed out the last line of the story to me.

"You see, Brenda? You see? God held Ron's hand then, and He still holds it now!"

Ron finally met Jesus face to face. Do those who go before us remember us in the face of all that glory? Do they care that we live here and they don't? Does the glory of God swell over them to such a depth that the past is of no essence? Does it matter?

No, because when we became Christians, we moved our first allegiance to God.

About the time of this accident, Ron started to collect eagles. Isaiah 40:31 became his favourite verse:

But those who wait for the Lord [who expect, look for, and hope in Him] shall change and renew their strength and power; they shall lift their wings and mount up [close to God] as eagles [mount up to the sun]; they shall run and not be weary, they shall walk and not faint or become tired.

As a result, eagle notepads, statues, and pictures graced our home. I put my foot down on the drapes. Picture our house as convocation of eagles amid a sea of green-and-yellow miniature John Deere equipment against sparkling blue walls, my favourite. Well, the blue walls did make a suitable background for the eagles!

Ron breathed as long as God ordained it. Like St. Paul, he "*fought the good (worthy, honorable, and noble) fight*," he "*finished the race*," and he "*kept (firmly held) the faith*" (2 Timothy 4:7).

If everything passes through God's hands first, that means Ron's death did as well. What a comforting thought! God experienced Ron's passing before I did. Surely that makes the pain less? How would I ever cope otherwise? Does that mean "Hey, Brenda, my princess, my honey, you can do this because God is going through every bit of it with you"?

New Resolve: Do not try harder but instead lean harder, on Jesus and the grace of God.

Fears are legion, a mob, really. Think huge crowds at basketball or hockey games. Think throngs of people watching a parade or the queen of England attending an event in your local town. Think Christians who know better yet still find

THE PREGNANT PAUSE OF GRIEF

themselves in this state, temporarily forgetting who they are in Christ.

Anyway, back to those fears. In all my life, I had probably spent less than two weeks of nights alone. The first time, Ron drove to a tractor pull several hours away. I stayed alone in our creaky old farmhouse with its share of critters and crawlers. Oh, none that you could see—just the ones in my wildly active imagination. Ask the kids about the day I saw a mouse. I corralled those teens with me on the stairs for hours till finally Ron came home and set a mousetrap. Sigh. *"For as he thinketh in his heart, so is he"* (Proverbs 23:7, KJV). (Read the whole story in *Meeting Myself: Snippets from a Binging and Bulging Mind*.)

Here are more thoughts on the same subject: *"All the days of the desponding and afflicted are made evil [by anxious thoughts and forebodings], but he who has a glad heart has a continual feast [regardless of circumstances]"* (Proverbs 15:15).

Oh.

We can ask God to remind us all over again how to take control of our minds and filter our thoughts. Maybe then, our stumbling will glorify Him.

Again I practice the pink elephant. Try it yourself. Close your eyes and see pink elephants playing tag on the plains of Africa. Watch those pink elephants tread water in the river. Observe them as they play catch with fallen coconuts.

Now, stop thinking of pink elephants!

Ha! Gotcha! It's impossible!

Now think purple polka-dotted giraffes racing across grassy slopes and sliding down mountains. When you do that, the elephants finally disappear.

Negative thoughts become obsessions that take over our lives. We can think pink-elephant fears or dwell on purple-polka-dotted-giraffe godly positive thoughts.

BRENDA J. WOOD

> *Summing it all up, friends, I'd say you'll do best by filling your minds and meditating on things true, noble, reputable, authentic, compelling, gracious—the best, not the worst; the beautiful, not the ugly; things to praise, not things to curse. Put into practice what you learned from me, what you heard and saw and realized. Do that, and God, who makes everything work together, will work you into his most excellent harmonies* (Philippians 4:8–9, MSG).

Fears abound in me when I let my mind wander. Does that happen to you too? "*Do not let your hearts be troubled, neither let them be afraid. [Stop allowing yourselves to be agitated and disturbed; and do not permit yourselves to be fearful and intimidated and cowardly and unsettled.]* (John 14:27).

Many folks try to avoid the flu by getting the flu shot, washing their hands to a couple of choruses of "Happy Birthday," staying away from crowds, and sneezing into their elbows.

Jesus describes Taadficu, a more deadly flu strain, in John 14:27. This virulent flu affects personal peace and occurs every time we forget to "*guard over [our] hearts and minds in Christ Jesus*" (Philippians 4:7).

Taadficu stands for "troubled, afraid, agitated, disturbed, fearful, intimidated, cowardly, and unsettled." Heart washing is the only cure. Symptoms show up when we don't lean on God. The more we practice keeping our minds on Christ, the more we avoid infection. That's more fun than vaccine shots, chapped hands, or even elbow-sneezing!

"Bet you can't read this correctly," laughed my friend.

It looked easy enough (Mr Ducks, Mr Knot, Mr Sew, whale oil bee, Mr Ducks). I read what I thought I saw. "Mister Ducks, Mister Knot, Mister Sew, whale oil bee, Mister Ducks."

THE PREGNANT PAUSE OF GRIEF

Grinning, she replied, "That's what it looks like, but it really says, ''Em are ducks.' ''Em are not.' ''Em are so!' 'Well, I'll be! 'Em are ducks!'" What we think we see is not what we see.

Swimming ducks paddle their little webbed feet furiously under the water. On top, our eyes only see large flocks of birds dotting the waterways. Which ones are really the ducks?

When we concentrate only on our troubles, that's all we can see. Right now my eyes see Ron's death and my widow status. When life crowds in an illness, family troubles, disease, loneliness, fear, dishonesty, murders, and war, who wouldn't get rattled? The part I can't see is so much bigger than my little reality. In the midst of these life issues, God is teaching willing souls to trust Him. I sure want to be one of those; don't you?

The fundamental fact of existence is that this trust in God, this faith, is the firm foundation under everything that makes life worth living. It's our handle on what we can't see (Hebrews 11:1).

Ron has a new career now. He's in the stands with the rest of those great crowds of witnesses, all of them encouraging us toward our best:

Therefore then, since we are surrounded by so great a cloud of witnesses [who have borne testimony to the Truth], let us strip off and throw aside every encumbrance (unnecessary weight) and that sin which so readily (deftly and cleverly) clings to and entangles us, and let us run with patient endurance and steady and active persistence the appointed course of the race that is set before us (Hebrews 12:1).

"Pack your oldest underwear," suggested my friend. "Throw the used pair into the hotel wastebasket. Your suitcase gets lighter every day."

Well, I just happened to be preparing for a trip to Israel! All my old underwear, the ones with stretched out elastic and faded colours, went into my bag.

Then I read Psalm 71:9. *"Cast me not off nor send me away in the time of old age; forsake me not when my strength is spent and my powers fail."* Thankfully, closer study revealed that the psalmist was speaking about himself, not my old underwear!

The first tossing was difficult, but I reasoned that I'd be in a new hotel the next day. Anyway, if the maid snooped, wouldn't it serve her right?

What a freeing experience! I got rid of stuff I no longer needed, stuff that only weighed me down. Wouldn't it be great to get rid of old sins as easily as old underwear? The Bible says we can. Get the wastebasket handy. Let's start throwing!

My thoughts turn to God. Wouldn't we like Him to take our weighty wastebaskets into His hands? That way we can more easily run this strange and peculiar race others call our "new normal."

Most of the Things We Worry About Never Happen

9

Let me tell you a few stories of how we met God. Honestly, you will wonder where on earth my mind has been in the last two months. I did tell you about that fog, right? Okay, enough then.

We've had people bring food to our door when we were eating our last dredges. (Dredges: the bits of stuff in the freezer that you continually move around but hope never to have to eat.)

I finally got a vehicle of my own, one that teenagers couldn't wear out! I really loved that little car. I was *not* thrilled when Mom and Dad arrived a few days later in their expensive new vehicle, a carbon copy of mine, except for the price!

Shortly after that, my car got rear-ended in an accident and died an early death. A friend suggested we pray for a new one.

Half-heartedly, I agreed. A few months later, Dad gave me that annoying car, handpicked by God—for me. We drove it for years and 360,000 kilometres, but it still looked and behaved like brand new.

No Stewing Necessary

We've always given 10 percent. It seemed a small detail.
We rounded up the numbers so our giving wasn't stale.
But then the church was building, and all were asked to do their bit.
The number God gave Dear and me caused us to have a fit!
It really would be a miracle. There's no way we could do it.
We could trust God for the bucks or huff and puff and stew it.
Well, now, we refer to the date we signed that "giving debt"
As one great blessing in our lives, for God our need has met.
Never once since we began have we suffered fail or doubt,
For God, in all His mercy, is working it all out.

That donation came to 25 percent of our yearly income, but we pledged it because God had made it clear that we should do so. The very next day we got a house repair bill that came to almost the exact same amount. It was forgiven under a home ownership bill in place at the time. So you see, I've no reason to fear lack of provision.

Can you stand a few more investigations with me? Tears abound today, but rain clears fog, right? I bet you're counting on that; me too.

Apparently, emotional tears have a different chemical makeup, including a natural painkiller that makes loss bearable. I don't know if they work on a sore finger or a bad back, but a saddened mind of grief? Oh yes. Thanks, God. What a great idea! Cry on, I now say, cry on.

Another of my loathsome fears is safety. Foolish, really, when Ron's handiwork made our little house so safe and peaceful. Ron can't repair my heart, though. Pieces of my heart remain displaced; others are missing. Only God can put me back together again.

Humpty-Dumpty Brenda
Brenda, Brenda sat on a wall.
Brenda, Brenda had a great fall.
All the king's horses and all the king's men
Couldn't put Brenda together again.

Brenda, Brenda decided to stand
And follow the King who ruled the land
'Cause only that King could give her grace
And help her through this difficult place.

Years ago, I learned to talk myself out of panic attacks. I might need that information again. Still, I haven't come to that yet. No point in even entertaining that thought!

I feared missing Ron, yet now I stand in the midst of that and survive. Whew! Part of me knows that I cope better than Ron would have. He didn't even like me to be away for an evening, especially near the end. If I'd died suddenly, the stress of all that on top of his health problems would have been too much for him to bear.

Then, of course, my usual fear of food showed up. As I write this, I discover new truth about my personal drug of choice, food. Yes, I fear food.

Well, that's the end of that. Why should an inanimate potato or slice of bread curl itself around my larynx and choke me? No, enough of that. I choose control over that right now.

However, I occasionally succumb to the lure of a sniffy whiff of chocolate or freshly baked bread. I've made decisions to eat based on unsubstantial things like that.

Do you ever do that? Make a decision to do something one way, but when the opportunity arises proceed into the craziness of earlier thoughts not based on facts? What a bunch of weenies we are.

You Can Cut Off Toxic Toenails; People Aren't So Easy

10

My friend wore her favourite skirt to work, but the skirt only fit if she wore her rubber girdle. During the day, the girdle ripped, and a large lump of flesh escaped that girdle and appeared at her side. She couldn't take the girdle off, because then she wouldn't be able to wear the skirt. She taped the reluctant undergarment together. We called that tape "duck" tape because if that girdle ever let go again, we'd all have to duck!

Have you ever been in the line of fire when someone lets loose with a string of angry words? Or have you ever been that person of weak "duck" tape? Here is the problem:

> *I said, I will take heed and guard my ways, that I may sin not with my tongue; I will muzzle my mouth as with a*

> *bridle while the wicked are before me. I was dumb with silence, I held my peace without profit and had no comfort away from good, while my distress was renewed. My heart was hot within me. While I was musing, the fire burned; then I spoke with my tongue* (Psalm 39:1-3).

The best solution is in Psalm 141:3. That's where David asked God to help him keep his mouth shut and his lips sealed!

None of us can tame our tongue or keep our mouth shut without God's help. (Check out James chapter 3 to see how dangerous our tongues really are!) Sooner or later, our true feelings pop out. Circumstances bring toxic people out of the closet of "respectability and love" they've been hiding in for years. The big question is, how will we respond?

I made sure that I forgave my toxics. I stayed spiritually clean before God. However, I never put myself in a place where they could attack me again. Don't fall for crocodile tears, either. The phrase *crocodile tears* stems from a story about crocodiles that pretended to cry, all the while luring their victims into eating range.

I add my fear of not being able to say no. The first few weeks AR were a whirl of forgetfulness. Without my journal I wouldn't remember anything that happened. I tried to follow the advice of a neighbour. He always said yes when anyone invited him to dinner. "If you don't," he said, "eventually, they stop asking you."

I made myself dizzy trying to keep up with the kindnesses of well-meaning folks. I attended boring business events that would have been better avoided. I entertained and fed more people than McDonalds. All it got me was tired.

Now I close the door and take a nap when I need one, make a coffee, and drink it in silence. Sometimes I haul out an easy-to-decipher mystery novel and pretend I don't have a clue how it ends.

This next one is as foolish as it gets. On a "poor me" day this thought crosses my mind: The family loved Ron more than me.

Now does that beat all?

I'm reminded of a mom who was asked which of her children she loved the best. "I love the one that needs me the most," she answered wisely. For several years, Ron needed the most.

We all wanted to spend as much time as possible with him. Each of us did everything we could to get that time. If, for the family, it meant hanging with Dad while Mom cooked, baked, and set out meals, so be it. If, for me, it meant giving up events and people I ordinarily enjoyed, so be it. We had some time but desperately craved more.

And you do too, though you might not realize it now. You want hugs more than candy, conversation more than television, and kindred hearts more than a paycheque. Oh yes.

For some time I feared displaying my grief in the wrong places and to the wrong people. I did mention the Toxic Togas, didn't I? Oh, maybe not the toga part. Toxic folks wrap themselves in what seems like a garment of mourning. If they happen to stand on the corner nearest you, the toga falls to the ground, and they share their splendidly naked version of your truth as they perceive it.

Maybe this explains it a bit better: "*Lord, how they are increased who trouble me! Many are they who rise up against me. Many are saying of me, There is no help for him in God. Selah [pause, and calmly think of that]!*" (Psalm 3:1–2).

Toxic Togas set you up for a "poor me" day. In no time at all, Poor Me feels worse. Eventually her thoughts turn to incidents that happened years ago. Moan, sigh, Poor Me! May the comforting Holy Spirit get a grip on us as we reread those verses.

"*Selah*"! "*Pause, and calmly think of that*"? Pause and consider! That we've been treated unfairly, that others caused trouble? Selah! Now we can justify our long-past circumstances. Hurrah!

Then we read the next verses. Oops! "*But You, O Lord, are a shield for me, my glory, and the lifter of my head. With my voice I cry to the Lord, and He hears and answers me out of His holy hill. Selah [pause, and calmly think of that!]*" (Psalm 3:3–4).

Hopefully, God long since healed hurts and won the war in our hearts, so why revisit the battlefield? God asks us to be realistic about our circumstances. Then He reminds us to calmly consider that He's in charge and also that He gives the victory. Selah! (Here it is again. Pause and calmly consider that!)

What's done is done. May we pause, consider our trouble, and move on to consider that God is our shield, our glory, and the lifter of our heads. Selah.

That prayer of Jabez keeps popping up in my brain:
Jabez was more honorable than his brothers, and his mother named him Jabez saying, "Because I bore him with pain." Now Jabez called on the God of Israel, saying, "Oh that You would bless me indeed and enlarge my border, and that Your hand might be with me, and that You would keep me from harm that it may not pain me!" And God granted him what he requested (1 Chronicles 4:9–10, NASB).

Don't we want God to bless us and expand our borders—unless that border is our clothing size? We yearn for God's presence to keep us from pain. We want to tunnel through the

THE PREGNANT PAUSE OF GRIEF

mountain facing us. What kind of pain do we want to get away from? Why, ourselves and our circumstances, of course! We want to abandon our flesh, the ungodly part of us.

Jabez was known as Pain, and I expect he lived up to his name. Don't we all? It's hard to get free from the stigma of the past. The world watches our label and expects more of the same. When Jabez asked God to keep him from pain, perhaps he too wanted to be free of his label. Maybe he wanted to expand beyond being a pain. Why wouldn't he want to escape that fleshly part of him that separated him from God? It's good to know that even when we have pain, we don't have to be one.

He's Not That Easy to Forget

11

Just when we investigate and deal with one fear, another pops up. Reminder to self: "*For God did not give us a spirit of timidity (of cowardice, of craven and cringing and fawning fear), but [He has given us a spirit] of power and of love and of calm and well-balanced mind and discipline and self-control*" (2 Timothy 1:7).

I got this notion that I was forgetting Ron, what he sounded like, how he smiled, and how much he loved me. One day, I glanced into our second bathroom, the ensuite, which Ron mostly used. He kept all his shaving bits in there, along with his favourite reading material, antique tractor magazines. I thought, *That is the last roll of toilet paper Ron ever touched.* I thought of ways to save it. Maybe if I never used that bathroom again, I could pretend he still lived here.

When I mentioned this to my walking pal, she grabbed me by the arm and turned us toward home. "You get in that house right this minute and get rid of that toilet paper!" she cried. I knew she was right, but in my head I was already creating "the shrine." I had visions of wrapping it in aluminium foil to protect it from wear and tear. Perhaps I'd tie the wrapping with a John-Deere-green ribbon.

Over the next few days that bathroom became a frightening place for me. In my head, I saw Ron in his last days, having to be in that room so much and getting weaker by the minute. I saw him sitting on his walker as I wheeled him there. The walker was too wide, or perhaps the door was too narrow. He'd struggle to stand up and move to the raised toilet seat. The walker had stood between us, a silent testimony to his failing strength and the fact that I could no longer help him in all the ways he needed.

Finally, I came to the conclusion that I had to redecorate that room. I refused to be afraid in my own home. First, the night light went. That light made my heart sad all through the midnight hours because Ron's suffering, weakened body seemed to be in my view all the time. I tossed the seat raiser. I didn't need it, and it just reminded me of the hip surgery that necessitated it.

I gave the miniature John Deere tractor Christmas lights to our youngest grandsons. When I handed all the tractor magazines to the three-year-old, he made his wishes clear. "Want green one!" he exclaimed. There's another born and bred green-and-yellow John Deere fan in the family. You gotta love it.

I'd made the curtains from a denim shirt of Ron's that got a little too small. By the end of his life, it would have swallowed him up. Of course it had John Deere fabric pockets. I generally made all Ron's shirts because most purchased shirts only have one pocket, and my pocket guy needed at least two pockets to carry all his stuff. I sewed extra pockets on this particular shirt, and what better colour? Sometimes I think John Deere might be making more money on fabric than on actual implement sales.

I found special keepsakes in those pockets. One contained Ron's first card from a little granddaughter, and the other, an anniversary card from me. Oh, I'd handed over many since, but he must have loved this one. The lines go something like this.

To my Ronald.
The first time I saw you, I knew. My heart told me you were the person I'd waited for. My life suddenly made sense. Every moment was in preparation for this one. You swept away my doubts and fears, gently replacing them with the most wonderful love. From the very first time I saw you, I just knew.
Love from your Brenda, your sweetheart.

Those lines tell our truth so deeply.

As a child, I used to dream of my perfect tall, dark, and handsome Prince Charming. He'd sweep me off the family farm to an exciting life in the city. He'd dedicate his every spare moment to me and our six wonderful children.

Then I met Ron, not so tall, but handsome in an Elvis Presley sort of way. Ron loved the outdoors, farming, grease, and machinery. I fell in love at thirteen, the first time I saw him, and long before he noticed me. He denied this, but I know better!

Our actual courtship began at the local Strawberry Festival. I was sixteen. Ron came into the church kitchen and turned to hand me a tea towel. Time literally stood still for both of us. He was twenty-six. Needless to say, my parents weren't pleased, but Ron was everything I wanted to be. Somehow I sensed that he would keep me safe. Ron was the first person I trusted with my abuse story. He's the one who held me after those frightening flashback nightmares.

Redecorating also meant removing that toilet paper. Anyway, what would the kids think after my demise if they found a roll of toilet paper wrapped in shiny Christmas foil? Of course, by then it would be packaged against dust. It might even have its own special niche, perhaps on the fireplace mantle. Seriously now, it could become grounds for committal to a long-term facility for those mentally losing it.

Once when Ron had car trouble, he placed a collect call to my parents because he needed a ride home. The operator asked my mom if she would accept the phone charges from "Ron."

"Ron who?" she cried indignantly.

We'd been married for eight years!

Needless to say, Mom never heard the last about that one! It happens to all of us. The face may look familiar, but the name will not come. Thankfully, I do remember Ron, and if my mind ever disappears down some long winding trail of forgetfulness, evidence shows that even in the worst of dementia people continue to hold on to their earliest memories. Anyway, we are in God's Book of Remembrance, and He never forgets any of us.

"*And if anyone's [name] was not found recorded in the Book of Life, he was hurled into the lake of fire*" (Revelation 20:15). We get into that book by confessing our sin and asking forgiveness for it. Then we ask Jesus into our life as our Lord and Saviour. He died to pay the price for our sin; He remembers names but forgets sins!

"FOR I WILL BE MERCIFUL TO THEIR INIQUITIES, AND I WILL REMEMBER THEIR SINS NO MORE" (Hebrews 8:12, NASB).

Cancer took Ron's life, but it couldn't take away his credentials as a loving husband and father, a special friend, a celebrated mechanic and fix-it guy. It couldn't take away his dignity, the respect he earned from his colleagues, or the love of his family and friends. Death is limited. It can't stop love or memories. It can't take the eternal life we'll spend together.

"O death, where is your victory? O death, where is your sting?" (1 Corinthians 15:55).

When Did They Ever Want You to Have a Bad Day?

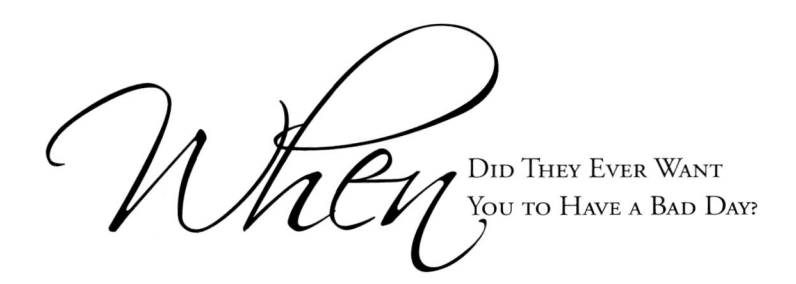

12

With emotion choking my voice, I could barely gasp out this sentence to my friend: "I had a good day today. Do you think that's all right?"

She stopped in her tracks and then pulled me to a halt. "Tell me," she cried out, "when did Ron ever want you to have a bad day?"

He never did. He wanted more for me than I ever dreamed for myself.

In our early years together, I once bought an orange plaid coat with our farm tax money. Yes, I was young and foolish, but the coat was on sale! I'm still sorry about that. Many a marriage has flown the coop for less.

What made the difference in ours? Yes, my hubby was tender-hearted. Yes, he loved me more than the tax money.

However, we had consciously decided never to consider divorce, ever. We were in it through thick and thin. Ron suffered through episodes like the coat while I suffered through episodes of shame and personal unforgiveness. In fact, I wore that coat to shreds for the shame of it.

I could continue with my list of personal failures, but if you had asked Ron who got the best deal in our marriage, he would have told you that he did. Go figure. That's what forgiving love looks like. Each one wills to forgive the other. Each one loves the other just the way they are…and helps them grow to a new, healthier place.

Without Ron's support, I wouldn't even have the career I have today. When I first saw the founder of Weight Watchers on TV, I determined that I too would help people be free of their food addictions. I dreamed of my own personal success in the fat game. I thought of places that needed a Weight Watchers class. I mentally listed all the friends and neighbours I'd like to take to class with me.

The trouble was, first I had to lose weight with the company. Then I'd have to travel to training sessions in the scary big city an hour's drive from our home.

I found the nearest class, about an hour away in the opposite direction. I coerced my sister-in-law and two nieces into going with me. I popped our two tiny tots in the car and drove to their town once a week. We gals would leave the children with my brother-in-law, and off we'd go.

When I started leaders' training, Ron would come home from a long day at work and drive us an hour into the scary city. The training began at 7 p.m. and often lasted till 11. The little ones, ages six and three, slept in the back of the car while Ron dozed fitfully in the front.

I've gotta tell you, there are no more stimulated talkers than

THE PREGNANT PAUSE OF GRIEF

a bunch of formerly fat people who've just found their tongues. We'd often blather on well past the official closing time.

Off we'd go home, and by 5 in the morning my honey would be back on the road at his current job, bombing sod onto people's lawns. Not ever did I hear one word of complaint.

Ron never made an issue of any of it. He just encouraged me to do my best. I discovered my joy and talent in writing. All that eventually led me to Stonecroft Ministries and a speaking career. Now I travel far and wide, sharing Jesus. I'm also back where I started, working as a Weight Watchers leader, and loving it.

That "good day" business reminded me of a movie Ron and I watched one day. I wish I could remember its name. This city slicker type guy visited a local farm, fell into the creek, and had his car attacked by a horse. Then pigs chewed him and a goat knocked him over. We laughed, and I said, "He's not having his best day, is he?"

By the end of the movie, the chap had married the farmer's daughter, made peace with the animals, and settled into the farm. It turned out to be his best day after all! Is it possible that our best days are still to come?

When circumstances look hopeless and unbearable, worry sometimes masks truth. Ridiculous fears bombard our thought life. Yet God continues to say, "By the end of the day, this will turn out for your good."

He promises! "*For I know the thoughts and plans that I have for you, says the Lord, thoughts and plans for welfare and peace and not for evil, to give you hope in your final outcome*" (Jeremiah 29:11).

And then He says it is possible to obey Him! "*Now what I am commanding you today is not too difficult for you or beyond your reach…No, the word is very near you; it is in your mouth and in your heart so you may obey it"* (Deuteronomy 30:11, 14, NIV).

That last verse startled me. God says, "Hey, whatever I ask you to do, it's not too hard!" (I'm guessing that statement includes this particular struggle we have!)

I made a list of a few things God has asked me to do in the years since I came to know Him personally. Some I instantly obeyed. Others I accompanied with a chorus of "It's too hard."

No doubt you, too, know the words to this song.

"It's too hard for me, Lord. Why don't you ask her? It's not fair to me, Lord; it isn't my fault." What a waste. Eventually I always gave in, and eventually I obeyed. In retrospect, it would have been far easier to just do the thing when God first asked me to.

So now if I ask why I am where I am, God's answer remains the same. "It is not too hard, Brenda. I am with you. You are not alone. I am not asking you to do anything millions of people before you have not had to do. You have role models. You have Me. What more do you need?"

No point in arguing with God! He is always right! To obey is not too hard. It will be worth it. And God has an answer for everything. *"I will [not merely walk, but] run the way of your commandments, when You give me a heart that is willing"* (Psalm 119:32).

For sixteen years, the last four as a Christian, I'd been the captive of an addictive food disorder called bulimia. I wanted to stop this vicious cycle of getting rid of my food after I ate it, but I just didn't feel that I had the power to do it.

Then one day, I suddenly realized I didn't want to live that way anymore. God had given me a willing heart! Though I've occasionally been tempted to fall back into bulimia, God's gift of a willing heart keeps me from slipping.

THE PREGNANT PAUSE OF GRIEF

You know, we could ask God for a willing heart to accept and, yes, even grow in spite of our circumstances. We could even ask for forgiveness for all that struggle we put in on our own when we didn't yet have a willing heart.

I think I'll add this postscript to my prayer: "Please, Lord, could my problem have a better name than *widow*?"

Lord Forgive Me When I Whine: I Have Two Feet; The World Is Mine

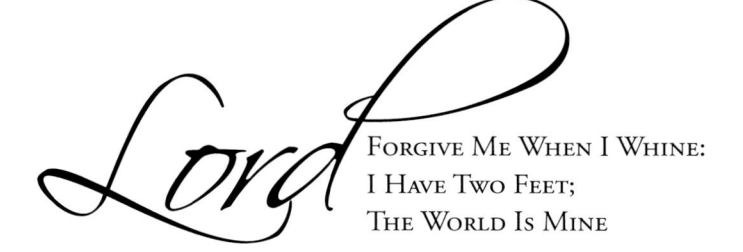

13

Ron never took walking for granted, because he'd suffered both a broken back and a hip replacement. He'd be all for my walking forward in this struggle of new normal.

Ron laid his body on the line for his family. He almost always worked at hard, physically intensive jobs. Oh, he occasionally took an inside job just so he could pay the bills. Still, his heart always yearned for a job involving either grease or fresh air, and preferable both. Those jobs wore him physically, but they also made him strong. He needed every bit of that strength toward the end.

Not one for wasting even a minute, Ron believed in working hard and playing hard. That's why he found it difficult to watch while others cut his lawn or raked his leaves. The biggest grin covered his face on those days he was well enough to haul out and use his own lawn mower.

So now, for the first time, dare I ask myself what the blessings might be in this new life? I fear the answers. Do they involve disloyalty to Ron because his absence makes them possible? No. That is not the way of God or Ron. I must learn to enjoy this season—at least I will when God gives me that willing heart we talked about.

"*I heard the voice of the Lord, saying, Whom shall I send? And who will go for Us? Then said I, Here am I; send me*" (Isaiah 6:8). When I first read this verse, I answered God just like Isaiah did. "Here I am, Lord. Send me." I saw my future as prophet-like, speaking Jesus into people's lives.

While I thought of speaking engagements and books, God had bigger ideas. "Here I am, Lord. Send me." And He did, into places no one wants to go—waiting rooms, CAT scan units, and operating theatres, into the valley of cancer scares and checkups. I didn't like it there. I wanted out.

I finally got it! Forget books and big public appearances!

I told God, "Here I am, Lord! Send me! To wherever you choose! Let my life speak Jesus into the lives of people who are in scary and difficult situations. Let them learn about Jesus and then choose to follow Him like I do."

Can I say I am still following Him now? Does being uncertain and afraid count against me? No, I don't think so. After all, legions of soldiers may be afraid, but they still follow their leader into battle. I'm following Christ because I have no other place to go.

Ron and I spent years in scary places. Known for his sense of humour and corny jokes, Ron spent his hospital time cheering up both patients and staff. I learned firsthand how a person stands in the strength of Christ, no matter what. Even now, I

THE PREGNANT PAUSE OF GRIEF

don't think of them as bad days. We celebrated every diagnosis with lunch, generally a Wendy's number 2 burger! No matter if it was bad or good news, we took it as from the hand of God. What if I apply those truths to my life right now?

Some time ago, some gals and I were on our way back to a hotel room after a day-long conference. One roommate scurried down the hall, way ahead of the rest of us.

"Hadn't we better catch up to her?" I asked.

"What for?" replied my friend. "She knows where we're going, but I'm the one with the key!"

In my heart, I know Jesus is the key holder, but my feet beg to differ. I run ahead of the key holder when I don't want to believe. I lag behind when I don't want to obey. I try to break down doors that only open when I let Him be the key.

I guess it takes some sore feet, tired bodies, and worn minds before we finally figure out that our personal plans have come to nothing. Only after we've stumbled and fallen or gotten stuck in the hallways of life do we finally figure that out. He is our key. Oh, that we would see Him as He is, the key to everything our lives should be.

My doctor says that grief is getting out of hand when we put things off, so she asks me if my taxes are done and if I pay bills on time. She doesn't ask me if I put the dishes into the dishwasher or vacuum the rug, and I do not volunteer this information. Secretly, I panic. Is that my grief showing? I vow to do better. After all, I have two feet!

Then I remember that I didn't like to do that boring stuff before Ron died. Maybe my issue is not grief recovery but total dislike of housework.

How Do You Eat an Elephant? One Bite at a Time

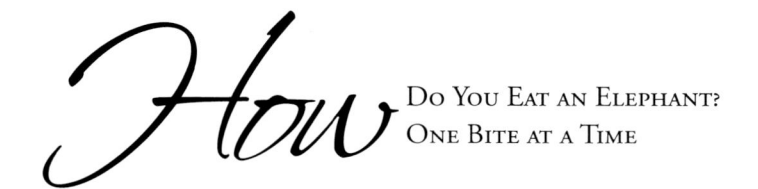

14

Even though we had lots of separate interests, Ron and I were one while we did them. Ron loved to play cards and fix things. Then, as now, I wrote, taught Bible studies, and worked for Weight Watchers. I'm also a motivational speaker.

When Ron felt better, he'd drive me to my speaking events. He'd have a meal somewhere, meet a new friend, and chat the time away. As much as possible, especially in our last years together, I chose my speaking dates to match Ron's free time.

Ron and I were stronger because we were one. We shared what had happened in our aloneness and together made decisions based on those conversations. Together was our favourite place to be. We were as different as night and day, but together we stood. Now I stand alone, but for the grace of God.

Our marriage wasn't supposed to make it. I was the Miss-Goody-Two-Shoes of the neighbourhood and Ron the Boy-With-A-Reputation! We married when I was eighteen and he a startling ten years older. We doted on each other and loved our way through endlessly difficult circumstances. We covenanted to never give up on our marriage. And we didn't. In the crunch of life, we were there for each other.

It would have been so easy to demand our own way, argue over petty things that didn't matter, or even hold grudges long after problems were settled. That is not God's way, and we chose not to make it ours.

Since he passed, I've heard this time and time again: "You are a strong, independent woman. You've always fought your own battles." In my head I hear, "*I can do all this through him who gives me strength*" (Philippians 4:13, NIV).

Nobody but me seems to get it. Ron was my strength and the wind beneath my wings. It isn't that we were weak when alone. It's that when we stood together, we stood as one with God as our third party. That love triangle made all the difference. God, Ron, and I connected as one and worked through our life issues together.

The Bible says that though one may be overpowered, two can defend themselves. A cord of three strands is not quickly broken (Ecclesiastes 4:12). I reminded God that He was the third person in our match. Then I asked Him how he felt about Ron's dying. God gently pointed me to the following verse: "*Precious (important and no light matter) in the sight of the Lord is the death of His saints (His loving ones)*" (Psalm 116:15).

I looked it up in other versions to be sure it wasn't a fluke:

Precious in the sight of the Lord is the death of his faithful servants (NIV).

Precious in the sight of the LORD Is the death of His saints (NKJV).
The death of one that belongs to the LORD is precious in his sight (NCV).

So then, every nuance of our life touches God! He understands our loss because He, too, lost a loved one. His Son Jesus died in a most terrible way. The great news is that Jesus didn't stay dead, and neither do our loved ones if they know Jesus as their personal Saviour!

"*O death where is thy sting? O grave, where is thy victory? The sting of death is sin; and the strength of sin is the law. But thanks be to God, which giveth us the victory through our Lord Jesus Christ*" (1 Corinthians 15:55-57, KJV). Losing our loved ones is hard, but God is grieving too. How cool is that?

Then God reminded me, "*Turn to me now, while there is time! Give me your hearts. Come with fasting, weeping, and mourning*" (Joel 2:12, NLT).

I decide to give God all my pain, every time it shows up. *Though the cherry trees don't blossom and the strawberries don't ripen, Though the apples are worm-eaten and the wheat fields stunted, Though the sheep pens are sheepless and the cattle barns empty, I'm singing joyful praise to GOD. I'm turning cartwheels of joy to my Savior God. Counting on GOD's Rule to prevail, I take heart and gain strength. I run like a deer. I feel like I'm king of the mountain!* (Habakkuk 3:17–19, MSG).

I took the time to rewrite this last verse to suit my circumstances, adding my name in place of the personal pronouns. It helped somehow. Maybe you'd like to do that too:

Though Ron will never come in the door of our home again,
though Brenda's heart aches with loneliness
and though Brenda's every meal tastes of sawdust and
disappointment,
though Brenda doesn't know whether Brenda's finances will
ever be enough or not,
Brenda is singing joyful praise to God.
Brenda is turning cartwheels of joy to her Saviour God.
Counting on God's rule to prevail, Brenda takes heart and
gains strength.
Brenda runs like a deer. Brenda feels like she is queen of the
mountain.

Are these statements true for us? Do our actions show our belief? Are we resolute of purpose? Will we do what it takes to be free? Does our desire match our obedience? Do emotions rule our hearts, heads, hands, feet, and health? Is our mourning becoming a habit? Is fear holding us back? Do we want to face our problems and get over them? If we do, are we forgetting? Do we really believe that we can do all things through Christ? (See Philippians 4:13.)

There was a certain man there who had suffered with a deep-seated and lingering disorder for thirty-eight years. When Jesus noticed him lying there [helpless], knowing that he had already been a long time in that condition, He said to him, Do you want to become well? [Are you really in earnest about getting well?] (John 5:5-6).

The King James Bible calls this fellow's illness an infirmity. The dictionary defines *infirmity* as weak, not strong, weak of mind, irresolute of purpose. Can lack of purpose keep a person stuck in one spot for years? Is it keeping us? Are we *stick* people? A *stick* person is a stuck person, full of himself; hence the "i."

Oh, if only we had grace to match both our desire and our obedience. That's one more thing to ask God for!

In Canada, we soldier on, driving in the most awful weather, ever hopeful of reaching our destination. Often a dusty white fog billows around our vehicles, clouding everyone's vision. Still, we drive on, because our goal is to get to that destination one way or another.

I blunder on, my heart and my tear ducts full of fog, because God's plan is supposed to mean healing and freedom. I may look funny while I travel, but I will arrive.

I am just like one of our grandsons, who crawled backwards for a few weeks but eventually figured out how to go forward at a mile a minute. Then he learned to walk by holding on to his parent's hands or the coffee table. He toddled, fell, crawled, got up, leaned on the couch, let go of his supports, and sometimes fell down. Then someone comforted him and wiped away his tears. Now he runs, plays sports, and rides his bike.

Even after a poor crop yield, my dad planted another crop the next year, because he knew from experience that eventually there's a good harvest. Surely God has upright walking and a harvest in mind for us.

We Change When We Live the Life We Never Thought We Could

15

Growing up, I sensed that others didn't understand my obsession with food; nor did they care to try. Chastisement for my overeating occurred on a regular basis, so eventually I took my eating underground. I ate normally in the presence of others but binged outrageously in secret. I even stole food if necessary, but that was pretty hard to do. Mom kept an iron hand on the fridge. She knew what was in there and who (out of six people!) she should call to accountability if anything was missing.

She had really good food-hiding places too. One Christmas, she made the best chocolate nut cookies. Soon, after my many bouts of nibbling, the whole jar disappeared. Where, oh where, did it go? I searched high and low, but no cookies for me.

A couple of weeks after the holiday, Mom reached up behind some tins in the cupboard. She hauled down that pretty clear glass jar with the red trim. The cookies sported green-grey fuzz. Because Mom never wasted a morsel, she was visibly upset. Frankly, I thought it served her right for hiding them so carefully.

I also learned something that fuelled my food fetish for years. A teenager never looks behind a can of vegetables for a sweet! I used my personal lesson to fool my own kids, thus saving all the special treats for myself.

Now my fridge is a foreign object to me. It does not do what it used to do. The margarine container stays full. I stopped eating butter and margarine years ago, in hopes of shrinking off a few pounds. Nope. Nada. Ron, on the other hand, stopped eating margarine only when he went up a few pounds. He'd give it up and within a week reach his optimum weight. Sigh.

Now, stuff is always in the fridge when I go back to use it. Sometimes it stays till it turns green. Then I have to throw it out. Like Mom, I do not like waste, but I don't yet have a knack for smaller batches. My recipes are beyond-belief size. I occasionally ask others to share a meal and, thus, help eat it up. But the other night I thought, *Am I missing someone to talk to, or am I missing Ron?* I recognized that having someone else in the house would not comfort me at all. I needed my Honey, but he wasn't there to eat scalloped potatoes and meatloaf.

It's been a week now, and those potatoes still sit in their tidy one-portion packages, waiting for someone to eat them. Methinks they wait in vain.

That doesn't mean I starve to death. Oh no, not by a long shot. Yesterday I didn't write one lick here, not one lick. I sat and read all day.

No, that's not exactly true. I sat and read and fed myself all day. None of it was worth the eating. When Ron passed, I gave away anything that didn't fit my weight loss plan…all the

THE PREGNANT PAUSE OF GRIEF

"good" stuff is gone. I binge on healthy food. Yippee? Not. I feel the intense guilt of the wicked, berating myself with continual mutterings and whines.

Yesterday, God got my attention about the whole thing, and I came to this conclusion: I ate because I was tired, literally bone-weary tired. Some days you have to go into your house, shut the door, and be alone with your grief. That's what happened to me, and in spite of the food—and no doubt the ouchy numbers at this coming week's weigh-in—I am the better for it.

As for not writing here, I weep my way though every entry. This is difficult, lonely, and exhausting. Add any other adjective you like. They'd probably all fit. I bet you feel the same way about your struggles.

God is faithful. He could protect us from eating ourselves to death. However, I expect He wants us to be part of the cure.

One of my fears AR is that I will eat myself into oblivion. What if I become one of those seven-hundred pounders who can't move out of their beds? God can help us with anything, but we have a part to play.

Wait a minute. That also means that in grief God can help us, but we have a part to play. Definitely worth thinking about and defining our roles more clearly.

My bleeding, broken widow heart screams, "Feed me!" What if we fail God by not walking in a way that glorifies Him? What if we fall flat on our faces again today? What if our binging never stops? What will we do? What if our love for God is not as pure as we would like it to be? What if this is more than we can bear, because we don't know or understand how to receive the grace God so freely offers?

Questions like these only pull us down into deeper depression. I struggle to remember that the Lord is my shepherd and that I can rest in peace, knowing I shall not want for anything. *"God, my shepherd! I don't need a thing. You have bedded me down in lush meadows, you find me quiet pools to drink from. True to your word, you let me catch my breath and send me in the right direction"* (Psalm 23:1–2, MSG).

So then, how can we move this promise from head knowledge into our hearts and our feet? Is it all about the asking? If so, we must ask our Shepherd God to help us choose to lie down in His tempting green pastures. Then we can ask Him to still the rushing waters of our riotous minds and fill us with Himself.

If you ask me for a dollar and I give it to you, you receive it. You might not spend it in the way I would choose, but I gave it to you. You have it. It is in your possession. You save it, spend it, or hoard it, but you still have it. Use it or not. You choose. You have it.

Now that we know what we have—Jesus, this great High Priest with ready access to God—let's not let it slip through our fingers. We don't have a priest who is out of touch with our reality. He's been through weakness and testing, experienced it all—all but the sin. So let's walk right up to him and get what he is so ready to give. Take the mercy, accept the help (Hebrews 4:16, MSG).

Our Giving God

Valentines of the world are fickle. They dwell
on external things
Like chocolate, lace, flowers, and expensive diamond rings.
The heart of God pours ever out the blood for which
Christ died.
He yearns to lavish that love on us and be our "forever" guide.
He pours out this attending love; His hope is ever thus:
That we would sense this God of Grace and ask Him to
belong to us.

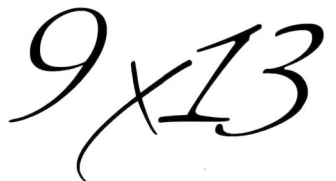

9x13 Baking Pans Scare Me

16

One of my first thoughts AR was that I wouldn't have the opportunity to make and serve large meals anymore. Poor Me thoughts like this ran through my brain: *No one will want to visit me since I am on my own. There will be no more friends and family to entertain.* I seriously contemplated giving away all my larger cooking pots and pans. I guess part of me thought I'd died too.

Yes, I know now that this was irrational thinking on my part. However, several gals told me their experiences, and I've since found it to be true. *His* family put up with you because you were attached. Now, he isn't in the mix. They don't have to bother about you anymore, so they don't. This isn't true of every relative of course. Most have a kind spot for you and continue to call, write, encourage, and visit.

A few married couples won't call either. People we'd known for almost fifty years suddenly vanished.

Are you now such a threat to the insecure missus that she won't be inviting you? That Christmas party you and your darling attended at their house for the last fifty years? Forget it. It doesn't say much for a union if a worn-out-from-nursing, beaten-down-by-grief, slightly older woman can steal a hubby. Now Elizabeth Taylor whisked Eddie Fisher into her boudoir, but for heaven's sake, it was Elizabeth Taylor, with diamonds attached!

It may help to take the missus aside and explain that you don't want her guy. While a few of my efforts in this area resulted in deadpan stares, you might have better results.

Of course, it is easier to seat a twosome to dinner. Still, I have difficulty understanding and accepting their discomfort. I guess when people don't know what to say to a grieving widow, it's just easier to take you off the guest list. That way, they don't have to see your sad face, and they can pretend that death will never interfere in their life plans.

As a rather cynical widowed friend said, "*Most guys our age aren't much of a catch. They have teeth and hair only because they bought and paid for them. They live on a pension, and someone monitors their pills. I do not intend to be a nurse with a purse.*" Let's face it. Women of our delicate age aren't beauty queens either.

Whatever you do, do not rush into dating and marriage. Let common sense be your guide. Of course, we are lonely, but we are lonely for the one person we cannot have. Nobody else can ever fill the spot left by our dearly departed.

Anyway, back to those large meals. I thought, *Who will visit me now? If they do, it will only be one or two or maybe three people at a time.* I fought this self-accusation by inviting folks over.

THE PREGNANT PAUSE OF GRIEF

Ron died on August 22. Our children and grandchildren came here for Thanksgiving as always. Our traditional turkey and stuffing came with tears this year.

The following Monday I invited ten ladies to eat leftovers. Our "aloneness" gave common ground. We were all so happy to have something to do that we put our best food forward. So there you are. My nine-by-thirteen-inch pans, the roasting trays, and the deep dish pie pans are still in use after all.

Another thought: it's a startling realization that everything "ours" is now yours. All those family letters and heirlooms, all the tools and motors, the yard implements, the car, the furniture, the investments, the house—all those things you once shared as a couple are now yours. With that comes the responsibility of care. Guilt accompanies the whole thing, of course, because you suddenly are responsible for twice as many things but have only half the monetary income. The thought is quite scary.

Ron knew how to fix things and make them last longer. He took care of the outside work and I the inside. As a youngster at home, I cut the lawn and worked in the fields, but when we married, Ron insisted that they would never be my jobs. He wanted me to sit in the house and sew a fine seam. He didn't actually say that, but he knew I'd sew a few fine seams, and all our clothes, curtains, and everything else besides.

He liked to bring me a rose whenever one bloomed on his little bush out front. I never picked them myself because I knew he looked forward to doing it. Peonies I'd take care of, but never the roses.

Just the other day, on the morning of November 10, I picked the last rose. November 10 may be rose season where you are, but it is definitely not so here. We've had a mild fall, but that rose just missed the first snowfall later that evening.

I stuck it in my mom's little blue rose bowl, and then I cried. I think of it as a gift from God to me, a reminder that my honey still loves me, even though we no longer live in the same season.

Before that, the three Rose of Sharon bushes bloomed weeks past their usual time. They wilted the week Ron passed, but the day after that they were up in full bloom again. Just try to explain that if you can. I can't.

That makes me think of how easily I fool myself into thinking Ron will be home any second. I mean, some days it feels like he hasn't left—that is, until some incident points it out to me all over again. Like just a minute ago. The car-repair people called and wanted to talk to me. The companies changed over the years, but for forty-eight years no garage guy ever wanted my opinion on anything except maybe what colour I liked and when we'd send the cheque.

And I find myself thinking how impossible it is that Ron is not here. How can this be? At times it is incomprehensible to me. At other times I take it in stride—well, more in limp.

Tender-hearted, romantic Ron scribbled little notes to me daily, mostly on those sticky-note papers. I'd find them tucked in office files, brief cases, books, or even a kitchen cupboard. I wish I'd kept more of them.

The poetry wasn't always the greatest, and sometimes the words were hard to decipher, but the heartfelt sentiment remained the same. Every woman loves a love note. I got more than my share, so I'm sharing them with you in the next chapter.

I Love You More Today Than I Did Yesterday

17

> Some ships have sails,
> some angels have wings.
> Some people have great bodies,
> that's what makes this rhyme ring.
> But God knew what He was doing
> 'cause He made you and me.
> Some will say that I am a torment.
> Some will say that I am a tease.
> But you will find no one better
> when you are in need.

NO TRUER WORD WAS EVER SPOKEN. IF YOU EVER NEEDED HELP to do something, my Ron was your go-to guy.

Just a Note
Just a note to say I love you. I really cannot count the ways. I love you more today than I did yesterday, but I will love you more tomorrow.

This next one he must have written when he realized how ill he was.
The notes I write, the notes you save,
will last you all your life,
but the ones I like to write are the ones
where I tell you that I love you
and am glad that you are my wife.

For our forty-fourth anniversary:
Dear Brenda, my love, forty-four years are here all ready, but it just seems like yesterday that I asked you to marry me. With all the bad thoughts that some people had and said that our love would not last, I wish they were around to see us now.

And this one:
To Brenda with love
The day was early, the time was now.
Showers of rain on the window made me lonesome for you.
Took pen in hand to write and say,
I love you in sun, rain, sleet and snow.
My love for you will always grow.

One favourite left Ron's pen on a "good doctor" day:
This is one Great Big special day as all my tests are great.
The only reason for that is God is so big and loving to us.

That means I love you more today than I did yesterday,
But I will love you more tomorrow!

And this one: *This note is just to say I love you and I will wait for your loving response in smiles or hugs or whichever comes first!*

Another, short, but oh so sweet: *Dear Brenda, You are the love of my life, my power and my strength.*

This one, written in 1994, just after our first grandchild was born, said,

Dear Brenda, I am writing just a small note to let you know that I love you and am very proud of you. Sometimes words do not sound right or express my feelings as well as a love note. When you do something special for somebody, it makes me feel proud that you are mine and mine alone. I want to thank you for your love and the pleasure of our four children, even though one is a grandchild. They are all special in my heart. [Note: the four children here included our son, our daughter, our son-in-law and our first grandchild. By the time Ron died, our family also included our daughter-in-law and four more grandchildren.]

Our forty-seventh anniversary brought forth this longer epic:

To the love of my life,
Hon, it may be forty-seven years as of tomorrow but right now it seems to be just like yesterday that you said that you would spend the rest of your life with me. I could not understand how a beautiful girl like you could love a strange dude like me. I am very proud to say that you are mine and I can love you with all my heart.

Forty-seven years seemed like a long time when we first got married but now it seems like yesterday that I said I do. In all these years, my love for you has grown stronger, through sickness and health. I pray to God each day to keep us both healthy and safe. When I look at you in the morning or at night I still see my beautiful girl of eighteen and my heart melts, and when you are away, it is so lonesome for me.

Lines like the last ones make me grateful that Ron is spared any more life challenges, physical or otherwise, especially the ones that leave you alone.

This one makes me cry: *Just look around the house everywhere and you will see me in all the little notes.* (And I do.)

This one was extra-special. I love it even more since I found the connecting verse in Ron's Bible.

My Special Flower
In God's garden where He grew flowers divine,
He grew a special flower, so beautiful, so fine.
He grew this special flower—
'Cause He knew it would be mine!

You see, I found the following jotting in Ron's Bible after he died. I'm reproducing it here as it looks on the paper.

STOP THIS TOP
LET ME OFF.
I'M TIRED OF GOING ROUND AND ROUND.
JUST WANT TO PUT MY FEET ON GOD'S GARDEN GROUND.

THE PREGNANT PAUSE OF GRIEF

My feet have a place on God's garden ground too. We will be together again some day.

Some of you are gagging by now because our love story is too honeyish for you. As great as my guy was, he wasn't the best husband ever. God promises that He, our Maker, is our husband. You can still catch the best one ever, just by entering into a personal relationship with God. All you have to do is ask.

"For thy Maker is thine husband; the LORD of hosts is his name; and thy Redeemer the Holy One of Israel; The God of the whole earth shall he be called" (Isaiah 54:5, KJV).

Heavenly Spouse
Some may not be so blessed
as to have a partner here,
But God has promised He'll be spouse,
to cherish, guide, and cheer.

Well-known elocutionist (and my mother-in-law) Clarissa Courtney Wood loved to recite lines from a poem she called "Are All the Children In?" (author unknown). The last stanza spoke of the children going to heaven and meeting Mother. Once again she'd ask, "Are all the children in?"

Grandma wasn't talking about getting us to bed before midnight. Like many mothers before and since, she yearned for her loved ones to ask Jesus into their life so that they would go to heaven when they died. She wanted to spend eternity with them.

"This is how much God loved the world: He gave his Son, his one and only Son. And this is why: so that no one need be destroyed; by believing in him, anyone can have a whole and lasting life. God didn't go to all the trouble of sending

> *his Son merely to point an accusing finger, telling the world how bad it was. He came to help, to put the world right again. Anyone who trusts in him is acquitted; anyone who refuses to trust him has long since been under the death sentence without knowing it. And why? Because of that person's failure to believe in the one-of-a-kind Son of God when introduced to him"* (John 3:16–18, MSG).

> *But whoever did want him, who believed he was who he claimed and would do what he said, He made to be their true selves, their child-of-God selves* (John 1:12, MSG).

> Are all the children in? Are you?
> *Here is the truth of the matter. Jesus is the Son of God. He came to earth as a babe in a manger—and He died on the cross just for you, just for me. He did that to pay the price for your sin and for mine. He was raised from the dead just for you, just for me. He's the mighty Son of God with the Holy nature of God Himself* (Romans 1:2–4, LB).

Nothing matters but Jesus and our personal relationship with Him. If you choose to say this prayer and ask Him into your life, then you too will have a personal relationship with Him.

> Dear Lord Jesus,
> I believe that You are the Son of God and that You died on the cross to pay the price for my sin.
>
> I believe that You rose from the dead and that You're alive right now. Please come into my life. Forgive my sin. Make me a member of Your family. I now turn from going my own way. I want You to be the centre of

my life. Thank You for Your gift of eternal life and for Your Holy Spirit, who has come to live in me. Amen.

Remember the date. Today you asked Jesus into your life, and today you begin to find out for yourself that Jesus is all there is and that Jesus is absolutely, completely, and forever enough!

Unexpected

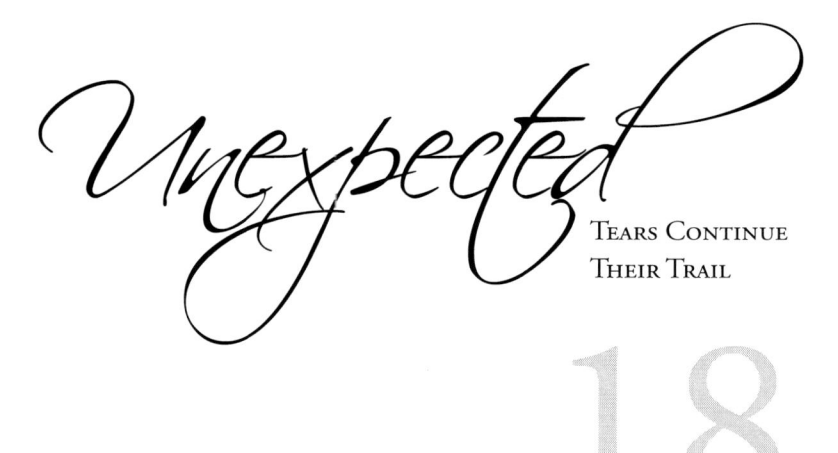

Tears Continue Their Trail

18

That wonderful movie *The King's Speech* spoke to my heart. The more the king tried to talk, the more he stammered, and the more he stammered, the more he couldn't talk. That's what fear does. Fear grabs hold if we don't keep our minds in a positive state.

Consider today. I rise early and get ready for church, confident I will not cry. I say to myself, *This is a good day. I won't weep all over everybody.* So sure am I that I go into the building with no preparation, no guard up against the simple, well-meaning question "How are you?" Everyone asks it of everyone, don't they? But the first person who speaks to me gets a gush of choking tears.

Where do they come from? Isn't there a reservoir in a person that eventually runs dry? If so, mine is in disarray, the taps are turned full on, and the plug is missing from the tub.

At first I plan to avoid all the places where I cry. Then I think, *How will I ever heal if I avoid the friends who love and care about me?* If I stop going to these tender spots, I'll lose my huge support system. What advantage is that? No, the tears must drip where they will.

What a silly statement! I can't make them stop, no matter what I do. Tears have a life of their own, and mine seem to have a longer lifespan than some.

Friends wrote comments like these after reading the last couple of paragraphs:

It takes time. With God's help and good friends you'll make it. If I was there I'd cry with you and we'd get everything flooded. Don't be hard on yourself. A loss of a dear one takes time. Real friends understand. Don't stay away, because sooner or later you have to face it. You wouldn't think twice about laughing out loud at something funny. Tears are just another emotion expressing feelings. Eventually you'll find yourself laughing more often than crying, but right now you are still healing, so let the tears flow if they must.

It's okay. Just cry; don't apologize. One day Jesus will wipe every tear dry, so find peace and rest in Him. Your tears are precious to us, and so are you. You allow us to walk beside you during these heartbreaking times, and I thank you for that honour as I read your blog and updates. We love you.

Tears are cleansing and perfectly okay. I love that you are so real about your journey with God and grief. You are a blessing to all of us. Tears are a language God understands.

Some people complained about my crying too much. I let them walk away. I stopped apologizing for my tears. God gave us the ability to cry for a reason. The way you share your grief in your blogs is inspirational. Anyone can build a brick wall around themselves for protection against emotions. It's those willing to face their emotions who are strong, and those who are willing to share them are even stronger. Thanks for sharing your tears with us. It gives me hope.

You know how many of us cried along with you at your loss. Seeing your hurt, and reading this post, I feel no shame or embarrassment; I only wish I could take some of that hurt away from you. Not a single person out there questions how you are grieving or the tears. Grieve. Hurt. Cry. Scream if you need to! You're never going to completely stop hurting, but the days when you feel like you can't get out of bed will get further apart. Brenda, you do *what you need to. People will respond to how* you *act and act accordingly.*

Then I read these verses:
[You should] be exceedingly glad on this account, though now for a little while you may be distressed by trials and suffer temptations, So that [the genuineness] of your faith may be tested, [your faith] which is infinitely more precious than the perishable gold which is tested and purified by fire. [This proving of your faith is intended] to redound to [your] praise and glory and honor when Jesus Christ (the Messiah, the Anointed One) is revealed (1 Peter 1:6–7).

Did you hear about the gal who lost her contact lens, prayed, and then found the lens only because it landed on the back of an astonished ant? I feel like her *before* she found her lens. I'm burdened by the surprise of Ron's death, even though it was expected. I've always strived to go through a problem, not deviated around it or over it by pretending it wasn't there.

A man was asked, "How are you doing?"

He answered, "Oh, I'm all right, under the circumstances."

His friend cried out, "What are you doing under there?"

Like the ant, if we take the time to look, we'll see Jesus magnified in the midst of our situation. May God give us the courage to stop living *under* our circumstances.

You might call me fainthearted, but only on occasion. It seems that I am trusting Jesus more than ever. Like the disciples, I have my good days and bad. I wonder if I should be telling you the truth of my life and have my doubts documented forever, like theirs. In spite of that thought I continue. Maybe this will never get published, and then it won't matter…

Meanwhile, the boat was far out to sea when the wind came up against them and they were battered by the waves. At about four o'clock in the morning, Jesus came toward them walking on the water. They were scared out of their wits. "A ghost!" they said, crying out in terror. But Jesus was quick to comfort them. "Courage, it's me. Don't be afraid." Peter, suddenly bold, said, "Master, if it's really you, call me to come to you on the water." He said, "Come ahead." Jumping out of the boat, Peter walked on the water to Jesus. But when he looked down at the waves churning beneath his feet, he lost his nerve and started to sink. He cried, "Master, save me!" Jesus didn't hesitate. He reached down and grabbed his hand. Then he said,

THE PREGNANT PAUSE OF GRIEF

"Faint-heart, what got into you?" (Matthew 14:24–31, MSG).

I ask myself, *Brenda, what on earth got into you that you doubted His presence for even a second?* Sure, I'm in my deepest water ever, doing the hardest thing I've ever been called to do. Yet isn't every new situation an opportunity to get closer to Jesus? He continues to stand in the midst of our deep, potentially drowning places, drawing us gently through the waves to Himself. He may find us in a fainthearted state, but He never leaves us there. What a relief! *"For the Lord sees not as man sees; for man looks on the outward appearance, but the Lord looks on the heart"* (1 Samuel 16:7).

It makes sense that if God wants to change our hearts more than anything, our hearts must be broken so He can repair them according to His standards.

Checklist
We are willing to be willing.
Jesus is standing near, ready to help us.
Will we cry out for Him, especially in our brokenness?
Then wait patiently while He helps us in His timing?

When I was expecting our first baby, "well-meaning" gals scared me to death with their personal birthing stories. Yikes! In the same way, I didn't fear a particular time of grief until others flood my mind with their grief stories.

"Now comes the most difficult part of the week, weekends alone."

"I can't stand eating alone. I cry through every meal."

"The first year is the worst."

"The second year is the worst. I'm just warning you."

101

"It's not so bad during the day, but the nights are terrible."
"Holidays are grim."

Thus, I suffered through Thanksgiving and began to fear Christmas. Ron and I shared bacon and eggs together first thing and then opened our presents. We didn't spend much but always made sure there were lots of little things under the tree. We enjoyed the rituals that made our day special. Now, new somethings take their place.

We made new paths when the children left home, and I know I will again. I just don't know what they will look like yet. It seems foolish to buy presents and pretend that Ron shopped for them. It's weird to wrap them and see them under the tree for weeks and then open them alone. Still, it may become my foolishness and my new tradition. It's too early to think about it and certainly too early to fear it. I did buy the fuzzy purple purse. When I'd mentioned it to Ron months before, he wanted to know why I hadn't bought it. Now I proudly use it and think of it as Ron's last gift to me.

As I listen to each widow's hard time and begin to add hers to mine, every day, all day, becomes something to dread. Is this really God's plan for us?

"A happy heart is good medicine and a cheerful mind works healing, but a broken spirit dries up the bones" (Proverbs 17:22). No, my goal is a happy heart and a cheerful mind, and less gloom and doom. After all, you can't give away what you don't have. If you are full of evil forebodings, worried about what might be, then you don't have a happy heart. *"All the days of the desponding and afflicted are made evil [by anxious thoughts and forebodings], but he who has a glad heart has a continual feast [regardless of circumstances]"* (Proverbs 15:15).

God stretches our faith like a rubber band, a too small pair of panty-hose, or the elastic on those old-fashioned suck-you-in

THE PREGNANT PAUSE OF GRIEF

undergarments. There's no point aiming for our original size. God won't let us go there. Imagine if He let go and we snapped right back to the beginning. Picture what happens when an elastic band is stretched beyond its original length. If you let it go, it sails through the air and lands in some hard-to-find place. Then you hunt for it, pick it up, and start stretching it all over again, until you get it where you want it. That's what God does with us. While we may slide back a bit, God just picks us up where we are and helps us move on.

I do not care to go through that major snapping again. It's too hard. Instead, I choose to move forward with God as He grows me past what I was into what I can become.

Fear Less and Become Fearless

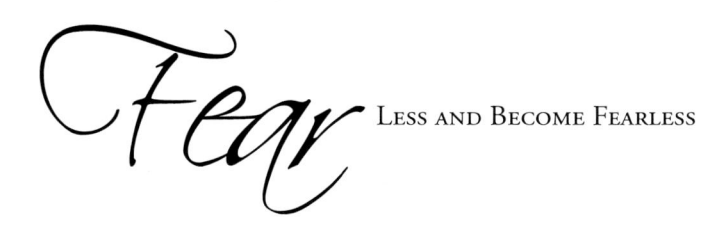

19

Many a time, I learned by experience that Jesus, the Son of God, who cared enough to die on the cross for my sin, also cared enough to take care of me—through my bad times as well as my good times.

What if I applied the lessons I learned from all those past challenges to this situation? Wouldn't the answers be the same? Wouldn't God still be faithful? Won't things get a bit better every day? Won't God continue to supply my need, just as He always has? *"My God will liberally supply (fill to the full) your every need according to His riches in glory in Christ Jesus"* (Philippians 4:19).

When we ask Christ into our life, He helps us to face whatever arises. *"Then Jehoshaphat feared, and set himself [determinedly, as his vital need] to seek the Lord; he proclaimed a fast in all Judah"* (2 Chronicles 20:3).

You might want to read the whole chapter for yourself. Jehoshaphat faced fear by seeking the Lord in prayer and calling on the community to fast. Here is the surprising thing: Lots of them showed up and did just that. They fasted and prayed!

I've been praying a bunch but not fasting so much. There's no reason I can't. I don't have to prepare meals according to anyone else's hunger schedule.

Judah praised God and admitted their weakness. Haven't I been doing that for the last several thousand words? God reminded them that it wasn't their battle to fight but His. Jehoshaphat said, "*We do not know what to do, but our eyes are upon You*" (2 Chronicles 20:12). Jehoshaphat did know what to do. He put his eyes on God. Eyes up, everyone!

God answered them with these words: "*Be not afraid or dismayed at this great multitude; for the battle is not yours, but God's…take your positions, stand still, and see the deliverance of the Lord*" (2 Chronicles 20:15–17).

And they did just that. They went out early in the day, trusting God. God won the battle, and His people praised Him and gave Him thanks.

I meant to do it weeks ago—that is, find things to thank God for in this new life. Why not make your own list?

Here is mine, so far. God provides me with enough to live on. I depend on Him. I wait with great excitement to see how He'll make ends meet this month. He always does. I continue to tithe, even if the amount is way less than it used to be.

I enjoy buying, preparing, and eating food that I really like. Some I haven't had in the house for years. Ron never denied me any of them, but a meat-and-potato guy likes meat and potatoes, so I always cooked that way. He liked pasta well enough, but it hiked up his blood glucose, so we seldom ate it.

THE PREGNANT PAUSE OF GRIEF

The children and grandchildren are supportive and loving. I try not to ask for much of their time or talents. I don't want to be one of those needy in-laws that demand everything and give nothing in return.

Ron picked our car repair people over the years, and the current ones have taken me on with generosity and kindness. "No question is too silly," they say. "That fellow, Ron, made us laugh just by walking in the door. We will take care of that car for you." And they do.

My time is my own. I write, take on extra classes at Weight Watchers, lead Bible studies to my heart's content, and occasionally eat supper early or late. I can sleep in, which I never did. I go to bed at eight if I want. It just occurred to me that since I sleep on only one side of the bed, next week I can switch to the other side. That way, I won't have to wash the sheets so often!

Comedian George Burns missed his Gracie terribly after she died. I once heard him tell an interviewer that when he couldn't stand it he slept in Gracie's bed, and that seemed to help. Worth a try, I think.

I keep busy. I pray for comfort, and when the Lord gives me songs in the night, most often they include this line: "Your grace is enough for me!"

I determined early on to ask God for scriptural experiences only. I told Him I didn't want any unheavenly manifestations. No essence of Ron sitting on the bed, as though he were still here with me. No sudden turning off of lights or disappearing or moved items. Jesus said there is no contact between the living and the dead (see Luke 16:26). I don't want to experience anything not true to His Word.

There's a story about a couple who were granted three magical wishes. They'd lost their son in some mutilating accident and were simply reeling with grief. They struggled with their wishes. I forget the first two—wealth or some such thing. Each secretly wanted the courage to wish their son back. Finally, the mom, in tremendous emotional agony, made that fatal wish. There arose a frightening gasp as the earth split and yielded up the boy from his grave. They heard a dragging foot, wails of pain, and more as their son returned, looking just as awful as when they buried him.

Why didn't they plan ahead? Why didn't they use the other wishes correctly? Why didn't they ask for the son to be healed, or else leave well enough alone? I prayed for DH (Darling Husband) Ron to be healed. And by God's grace he was, but not in the way I expected. No more pain, suffering, or sorrow. Right now, he shakes hands with all those who went before and sits on God's lap, soaking in God's love and enjoying God's best for him.

Oh, I pray for the courage to ignore my fears, to stop putting all my attention on them, and the wisdom to put my mind on Christ.

Dear readers, you didn't really know me before, because I wouldn't let you. Dregs of sexual abuse kept me penned up (no writing pun intended!) and unable to feel anything. Fears come from my old head, but I'm glad that now I have a heart that really feels emotion.

"But, after all, brains are not the best things in the world," said the Tin Woodman.
"Have you any?" inquired the Scarecrow.
"No, my head is quite empty," answered the Woodman. "But once I had brains, and a heart also; so, having tried them both, I should much rather have a heart."
L. Frank Baum, *The Wonderful Wizard of Oz* (Chicago: George M. Hill Company, May 17, 1900).

The Holy Spirit, the Word of God, and common sense must take hold. Emotionally, I desperately miss my darling. When I am able to think rationally, spiritually, I ask myself if I would want him here to suffer more. No. Would I want him to endure this all-consuming aloneness? No, absolutely not. Will I trust God to comfort and help me? If I don't, how will I dare call myself Christian?

And He said to them, [Why are you so fearful?] Where is your faith (your trust, your confidence in Me—in My veracity and My integrity)? And they were seized with alarm and profound and reverent dread, and they marveled, saying to one another, Who then is this, that He commands even wind and sea, and they obey Him? (Luke 8:25).

SINCE GOD
Since God commands the wind and the sea,
Then God, may You take command of me.
I'll do what You say. I'll go where You go
For no other reason but that You said so. Amen.

86 — Something Previously O.K. Becoming Not O.K.

Today no words come to my mind. Self-exposure hurts. I dare not write if I plan on going out in public later, because tears cascade down my cheeks with every word. After I leak all over the computer keys for three hours, my face is a blotchy blob of red sogginess, my state easily recognizable. This makes many people uncomfortable. They cope by avoiding the tears and, hence, also avoiding me.

Others more than compensate. They go the extra mile and weep all over me. This results in my sobbing all over again. Sigh. There is no pleasing a mourner.

Anyway, there is no danger today, because I can't think of anything more I want to say. Ron and I shared lots of untold private moments, but do you need to know them? For that matter, do I want to share them? Shouldn't some small part of Ron remain mine and mine alone?

I ask God for help. And He shows up like always, speaking through His Word.

"Lord, what shall I write about today?" I query.

And He drops these three little words into my heart: "Not a word."

"That's not funny, Lord," I sass back.

Oh oh.

Herod was delighted when Jesus showed up. He had wanted for a long time to see him, he'd heard so much about him. He hoped to see him do something spectacular. He peppered him with questions. Jesus didn't answer—not one word. But the high priests and religion scholars were right there, saying their piece, strident and shrill in their accusations (Luke 23:8–10, MSG).

Today, I'm Herod's first cousin. I want to see Jesus on my terms. I want my tears stopped and my heart healed. I demand miracles in my time zone, not His. I told you I expected to remember my own name by the end of three months of grieving. A pregnancy doesn't even show in the first trimester. What if the whole process gets worse? This last statement might mean that the rest of my senses aren't speaking with a full flame either, just a weak, wispy flicker.

Perhaps I should listen for God's voice with more intention, while ignoring mine as much as possible. Silencing my voice completely might be a better idea. So I sit here quietly pounding on computer keys with no thought but to let God guide the message. This chapter might be a doozy, because God always shows up big-time.

Witness the first verses of Psalm 86:

Bend an ear, GOD; answer me. I'm one miserable wretch! Keep me safe—haven't I lived a good life? Help your servant—I'm depending on you! You're my God; have mercy on me. I count on you from morning to night. Give your servant a happy life; I put myself in your hands! You're well-known as good and forgiving, bighearted to all who ask for help. Pay attention, GOD, to my prayer; bend down and listen to my cry for help. Every time I'm in trouble I call on you, confident that you'll answer (Psalm 86:1–7, MSG).

David, the author of Psalm 86, demanded that God answer his prayer. We both tell God how miserable we are, reminding Him that He owes us because of our faithfulness. We try to guilt God into showing up. We demand that God give us our version of a happy life.

"Pay attention, God!" we shout. "Get Yourself down here and listen. We're in trouble, God, and we need You *now!* So there!"

"P.S. God, show up now!"

What audacious behaviour! Are you an eighty-sixer too? Come on, tell the truth! You've had your life turned upside down. I know you have. Aren't you grateful that God listens and hears our heart cry when others have long ago tired of it?

Other phrases from the psalm catch my attention. "*God, you're the one, there's no one but you! Train me, GOD, to walk straight; then I'll follow your true path. Put me together, one heart and mind; then, undivided, I'll worship in joyful fear*" (Psalm 86:10–11, MSG). Who doesn't need training to deal with their current state of affairs? I sure need new skills to live out this "widow's walk" thing. Did you know that *widow's walk* is a term used to describe balconies on the top of seaside homes? A lonely wife would stand there, gazing into the distance, all the while hoping and praying for the return of her seafaring hubby. If he didn't come back, she walked that walkway alone, forever.

If I clung to the hope that Ron would come home any minute, what good would that do for me or anyone else? No, my widow's walk must move me forward. I am Humpty Dumpty. All the king's men can do nothing for me. God must put me back together again. My heart is in one place, my mind in another. I need the Lord to do surgery on me, to operate on me, so that my divided self gets back together again.

I know these next lines to be completely true: "*You've always been great toward me—what love! You snatched me from the brink of disaster!*" (Psalm 86:13, MSG).

And these speak volumes: "*God, these bullies have reared their heads! A gang of thugs is after me—and they don't care a thing about you*" (Psalm 86:14, MSG).

Toxins abound. Some are people and some are circumstances. Like the old saying goes, you can pick your friends but you can't pick your relatives. But this is also true: You can pick your attitude. I determine to be like God in this. He even tells us how.

"*But you, O God, are tender and kind, not easily angered, immense in love, and you never, never quit*" (Psalm 86:15, MSG). Don't you, too, want to be tender, kind, not easily angered, immense in love, and most of all, never quit doing the right, the godly, thing?

David begged God to look him in the eye. Not all of us dare to look anyone in the eye. Shame, fear, anger and other emotions keep us keeping our own counsel. Not good.

"*So look me in the eye and show kindness*" (Psalm 86:16, MSG). I love how David asked the same thing that I ask for every day and that I thank God for every night. I beg God for strength every morning. At night, I whisper thanks that together God and I made it through one more day.

THE PREGNANT PAUSE OF GRIEF

If it weren't in Scripture as a precedent, I don't know if I'd ever dare pray the next lines: "*Make a show of how much you love me so the bullies who hate me will stand there slack-jawed*" (Psalm 86:17, MSG). What a relief! God takes care of our toxins and gently, powerfully, puts us back on our feet. What a powerful revolutionary prayer if we but dare to pray it!

As a new Christian, I was afraid to pray unless I followed some "standardized" method. If I didn't adore God first, maybe He'd be angry. If I prayed out of sequence, maybe He wouldn't hear. This resulted in my not praying very much at all. Thankfully, there stands Psalm 86 and David, who let God know what's what right off.

God knows that our world is topsy-turvy. He recognizes that our heads are not where they should be. He knows we may do strange, unexplainable things.

The other morning, I looked for the outfit I thought I'd put into the laundry basket the night before. Some of it was there, but my underwear graced the shelf in front of the television. Surely I didn't put it there? What was I thinking? And why didn't I notice it when I turned on the news?

The answer is that I wasn't. Thinking, that is. I let my past and my future interfere with my present. I need to learn my own name and so much more.

Do What You Can and Let God Take Care of the Rest

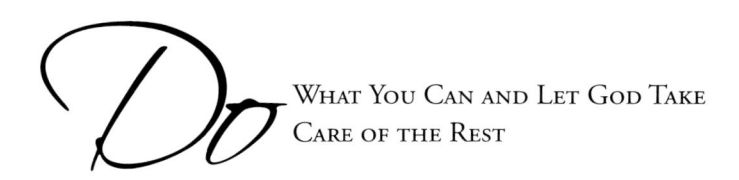

21

Several sites popped up when I googled "How did Moses feed the Israelites?" According to the calculations of people much better at math than I am, Moses needed about fifteen hundred tons of food and at least four thousand tons of firewood every twenty-four hours.

Keeping the Israelites watered and washed required about fifty million litres of water daily. To get them across the Red Sea in one night, he had to form them into a line more than three miles long. That means the "road" they travelled through the sea had to be at least three miles wide. Whew! How did Moses do it? Read the book of Exodus for yourself. Moses trusted God. "*By an act of faith, Israel walked through the Red Sea on dry ground. The Egyptians tried it and drowned*" (Hebrews 11:29, MSG).

Moses did what he could and believed God for the rest. *"The people who know their God shall prove themselves strong and shall stand firm and do exploits [for God]"* (Daniel 11:32).

So what needs are there in this little home now? It's been almost three months since Ron's death, and I still don't know my monthly income. The government continues its governing pace. It takes effort to trust God for my needs, even though Ron and I always lived that way. Well, we lived that way after we asked Jesus into our lives.

As a couple, we found it exciting to watch for and then see God act. The only difference between now and then is that Ron had at least half the faith. Now it's up to me to trust and believe. Perhaps God had purpose in Ron's passing? God is giving me the opportunity to grow my own faith in certain areas.

Does my home need less loneliness? God is a faithful companion. I am alone but not lonely. Do I need more comfort? The Holy Spirit, the Comforter of all comforters, lives here.

What if we applied Moses faith to our lives? What if we asked God for provision and expected it? What if we asked Him to meet our needs again… and again…and He did? Just because He does.

Moses' faith reminds of my cheese-and-onion pie recipe:

> Toss four cups of chopped onions with four cups of grated cheddar cheese. Pack the mix into a deep pie plate lined with pastry. It will be very full. Pay no attention. Stick all the mix into that pie shell. Add a top crust, pierce it, and plop it in the oven. Bake at 425 degrees F. for ten minutes and then 350 degrees for another 30–35. Serve it hot or cold. Yum! Serving a crowd? Use a 9x13" baking dish (without fear).

THE PREGNANT PAUSE OF GRIEF

No one believes that the only ingredients are cheese, onions, and pastry. "Haven't you forgotten something?" they ask.

I invite you to try my pie recipe and my God, and then let Him try you.

Moses' faith actively takes over my life. For instance, I had to cancel evidence of my Honey's life because powers-that-be demanded that proof of Ron's existence be erased from the books of the world. Both they and the funeral home tried to make it as painless as possible, but the world of paper waits for no man (or woman). Papers must be signed, health cards and licenses cancelled, and pensions reorganized.

I filled out and delivered the forms alone, not because I'm some sort of spiritual warrior but because Ron's life was personal and private. He deserved my personal, wifely touch, and I saw it as my last chance to do something for him. Warning! It makes for intense pain. Until that paperwork attested to Ron's death, part of me could pretend he was not gone.

Do you sense a recurring theme here? A friend says her worst day was the anniversary of her hubby's death. A whole year of pretending, and the truth finally hit her like a ton of bricks. Ouch. Still, I continue to pretend sometimes. I find it quite comforting, though not the least bit sensible.

On paper, Ron is past tense. He used to need health insurance, a driving license, a passport, and a social insurance number. In my heart he lives in the present, but I occasionally find myself hanging out in Nazareth. That's how I describe my unbelieving self. Read Mark 6:1–6 for yourself. Verses 5 and 6 are especially telling.

Jesus couldn't do any miracles in his hometown, because the people didn't believe. They saw him as just one of the local boys, and because of that they stumbled and fell. Jesus was amazed at their lack of faith (Mark 6:6).

We amaze Christ daily with our lack of faith. The only thing more awful than the things that happen to us is what we do with them. We may go to church and even quote Bible verses, but when we don't believe in or trust God we are citizens of Nazareth, at least part of the time. We don't always believe God 100 percent, especially when times are tough. We pick and choose the parts of God's Word that we like. We whine when trouble hits.

"But Jael, Heber's wife, took a tent pin and a hammer in her hand and went softly to him and drove the pin through his temple and into the ground; for he was in a deep sleep from weariness. So he died" (Judges 4:21). Jael likely hammered in tent pegs every day of her adult life. She learned to serve her Father God by doing what she needed to do, with what she had on hand, every day. She faced the life God gave her and conquered her personal enemies.

Now what have I done for years? I've followed the leading of the Christ. I followed Him when the rest of the family thought I was over the edge. My immediate family came to faith in Christ shortly after I did, but in the meanwhile they thought it just more craziness from their bulimic wife and mother.

This is the same woman who decided we should walk along a bush wilderness path right after church, dressed in suits, high heels, and frilly blouses. This is the same woman who made her teenage children cower on the stairs with her for a complete day after a mouse made a three-second appearance.

When my immediates came on board, the extended family really started raising their collective eyebrows. It was a furious time of self-defence and God defence, until we figured out that God could defend Himself and us too. What a relief! All we had to do was follow the path He'd laid out before us. So we did.

THE PREGNANT PAUSE OF GRIEF

I thought about life issues stemming from my food addiction and my weight. I was the kind of gal who ate three Christmas cakes in one season, one slice at a time. This left us without Christmas cake for the actual day. You know slivers of food have no calories, right? I spent all my energy and resources trying to make my outside look perfect. January after January and diet after diet, I moaned my way through my life. No diet had the desired results, because food was the symptom of the real problem.

Thankfully, somebody told me about Jesus. All I had to do was turn from my old life, ask Him to forgive me, and ask Him to come into my life. I did that very thing, and my life certainly changed for the better.

I'm grateful for lessons learned in hard places. God is faithful in both the good times and the bad. When the way is rough, our faith has a chance to grow. Our path might not be our favourite, but God allows us to have it.

Christlike living is a learned way of life. Any idiot can face a crisis. It's the day-to-day living that wears you out. I pray it won't get me.

The world moves; so do we. Fog lifts a bit. Why be surprised? That very same God who brought lessons years ago is the God of today. May we always fight the good fight, finish the course, and keep the faith. (See 1 Timothy 4:7.)

Having Said That...

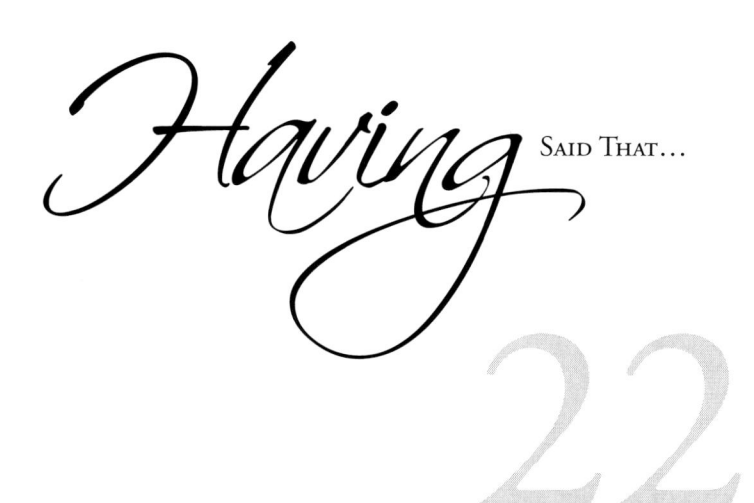

22

*I'd rather be a could-be if I cannot be an are;
Because a could-be is a maybe who is reaching for a star.
I'd rather be a has-been than a might-have-been, by far,
For a might-have-been has never been, but a has was once an are.*
Milton Berle (otherwise known as Mr. Television)

On August 20, 2011, Ron and I were together in our little house. The family brought lunch. Ron rested. The grandchildren played high-spirited games around our feet. All of this was familiar, but now Ron rested in a hospital bed, on morphine for pain and seldom conscious. The grandchildren gazed at Afi (Icelandic for *Grandpa*) and said, "Afi sleeping. Night, Afi." Then they continued to play, trusting and expecting their parents to keep things right.

The adults cried some, reminisced some, feared some, while the grandchildren simply accepted and trusted in their parents' love. In time, the rest of us would remember that we are loved. We know Jesus. We have right relationships with God. We eventually determined (all over again!) to trust Him. This seemed distant for the time being. Still, deep down, we knew that God makes all things right, even when everything seems so wrong.

Most "widow" books share one common denominator. There is no right or wrong. Your grief is yours and yours alone. Don't let anyone tell you what to say, how to behave, when to go back to work or take off your wedding rings. Don't let anyone tell you when to stop crying.

Press your tongue against the roof of your mouth. Pinch your finger till it turns blue; feel that pain instead. Bite your lip. Oh, yes, I know and have used all those tricks at various times in my life, even on the speaker's platform. Now, somehow they don't seem to work so well. Tears keep leaking out. Let's accept them for what they are: healing.

So if you see us crying, please pat us on the shoulder, hug us, or tell us you pray for us. Definitely invite us for coffee, but never tell us to stop crying. If we could, we would. We do not like making spectacles of ourselves in public any more than you like to see it.

If we know Jesus as our personal Saviour, we are "ewe-nique," one of a kind. Jesus doesn't carbon copy His sheep, so it follows that even our grief processes will differ. People who criticize that fact also will criticize a hundred other things when they get the chance.

Don't think that grief protects you. With your spouse gone,

THE PREGNANT PAUSE OF GRIEF

a few people who wanted to tell you off before and didn't feel free to do so will now. Don't fight it. Instead, take it to God. Refuse entanglement in other people's barbed wire.

Early on in Ron's illness, he decided that he didn't want the world to know how sick he was. I became his protector, just as he had protected me for so many years. The phone would ring, and I'd ask him if he wanted to talk. We didn't have call display, so it might have been the furnace man or the next-door neighbour on the line. No matter. Ron based his decision on his energy level that day.

The same was true of visitors. If he couldn't cope, he'd go lie down. I'd fend them off.

A few took offence. They wanted to talk when they wanted to talk, and that was that. They neither knew nor cared that their calls and visits drained Ron. They only cared to have their needs met.

I've always been a "yes" person. I've given over my own power to others forever. I do not like to cause a disturbance. But this was about Ron. It was what he wanted, and I wanted to give him what he wanted. Isn't that part of love? If we'd been in the opposite place, I'd likely have dragged myself to the phone, listened through endlessly boring conversations, and generally put up with it all. But this was not about me.

Eventually we take a position because it's the right thing to do. So I stood against considerable opposition. Even now I continue to take blows for that. I expected to take flack for it, but I'm surprised at the attitude of those who do not care to understand that this was Ron's last wish. He asked for peace and quiet, and I helped him get it.

Hubby works late, and wife shushes children so he can sleep in. Or maybe he finally gets an afternoon nap, and so she herds the family to the backyard. A teenager may not be at her best of a morning, so the family whispers through the early hours because it means peace for everybody.

Moms tiptoe through life for the sake of their families. We get up early, quietly shower and sip our coffee. This silence becomes our way of life.

When Ron and I moved to our little downsizing home, I continued this habit. Ron seldom slept through the night, and I've always been an early riser. I made coffee by the light of the fridge door so the overhead kitchen light wouldn't glare toward the bedroom and wake him. I sometimes read by flashlight. I took a shower after he awoke. I set the TV to mute and read captions on the screen. I kept the ringer off on the bedroom phone, turned down the living room phone, and even closed the windows against traffic.

Today I slammed a cupboard door by mistake…and listened for Ron's feet to hit the floor in the bedroom. I feel my loss in a new way because now silence doesn't matter. I guess it's okay, then, to cry out loud, "God, when everything feels so wrong, how can anything ever be right again?

For years I stifled my emotions, but now I don't know how to turn them off. Forget? Why would I want to? If I forget my honey, then I forget the years we spent together. I'd be calling those years meaningless. I would negate the very lives of my children and all our descendants to come.

How could I forget myself? How could I ever forget that Ron's tenderness and care helped me recover from the sexual abuse that choked my soul? How could I push away his essence? He concentrated his earthly love on me. Why would I even consider forgetting all the sacrifices he made physically, mentally, emotionally, and spiritually for me?

I've heard that if we step out in the world for the Lord, our family will be attacked, so I asked Ron this question a

THE PREGNANT PAUSE OF GRIEF

few months before he died: "Honey, you have been through so much. Maybe if I wasn't in the forefront, speaking for the Lord, you might not have had to go through all this pain and suffering. Would you change all that? Would you go back and wish me not to have done this?"

He didn't hesitate for a minute.

"No, absolutely not," he said.

If anyone deserved heaven (and none of us do), Ron did. When our church elders came to the hospital to pray with us before yet another medical test, they prayed for healing, comfort, and God's grace. Ron simply thanked God. In the midst of everything he experienced and continued to go through, he just thanked God!

Some folks took to calling him Job, in jest, I'm sure, but there was some truth in that title. Ron suffered so much *and yet* still stood for God. God restored everything in double measure to Job, and now Ron experiences the same. He's experiencing his rewards right now, in heaven.

Oh, and about that "thank you" business? You never have enough thank-you cards. Someone gave me three packages of cards just before Ron died. Privately, I thought, *When will I ever use these?* It turned out that I needed to buy lots more. I used all of the cards the funeral home gave me, and then I even had to make some.

At first, cards and letters, casseroles and flowers poured in. Bits of gift money over that first month made living possible. Phone calls never stopped. People dropped in simply to give hugs. They made financial donations to our church or to the cancer ward at our local hospital. Long-lost friends reappeared. Someone cut our grass; others covered for me at work. Someone lowered the flag in our yard to half-mast.

"What is that you have in your hand?" asked God.

And people answered him with their talents of giving, baking, writing, thoughtfulness, and encouragement. They cared about us more than they cared about themselves. They took the gift God gave them, and they gave it to us. They didn't just talk the talk; they walked the walk.

No one expects a thank you for a card, but I did thank all those who went out of their way to befriend us, including the funeral home and all those who took part in the service. Those people loved Ron too. Their hearts hurt. While they didn't know him in the same way I did, the life that they shared with Ron is over. Their comfort comes when I let them help me. That is hard for me to do, but I made a list of the things I needed, prayed over them, and asked Jesus to help me. I've actually been able to ask people for help. When they offer it, I take it.

As I said, our neighbour used to say that if people ask you to go somewhere you should always say yes. If you don't, they stop asking. So I say yes a bunch, even though I occasionally negotiate a change of date or time.

About four to six weeks after the loss, the cards and letters abruptly stop. To us, it may seem that they all stop caring, but that's not true. People have their own lives. They move on, and, I expect, they think we have also. That's because they have not shared our kind of loss.

There are those who know better. Some who have experienced this phenomenon will continue to remember you with cards; a few faithfuls phone. Oh that we would remember what it feels like to be abandoned! Now that we know better, we can be the ones who continue to phone, write, and visit those suffering like us. After all, isn't that the whole purpose of learning?

A Leap of Faith Is Just That

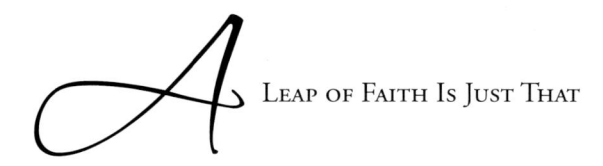

23

This morning, while I was reading my Bible, I asked God for a word to cling to for the day. Acts 3:1–13 grabbed my attention. Just so you know, I didn't hop all over the pages trying to find something to cheer me up. I simply started to read where I left off the day before.

Anyway, Peter and John were going to pray at the temple, but this crippled beggar guy lay right in their path. The beggar did the only thing that he knew how to do. He asked them for money. Peter told him they didn't have money, but they'd give him what they did have. In the name of Jesus, he demanded that poor fellow get up and walk.

Peter grabbed the beggar by the *"right hand with a firm grip and raised him up. And at once his feet and ankle bones became strong and steady, And leaping forth he stood and began to walk, and he went into the temple with them, walking and leaping and praising God*" (Acts 3:7–8).

Everybody recognized him as the guy who spent his time begging at the gate, but now they saw him walking about and praising God. The Bible says, "*They were filled with wonder and amazement (bewilderment, consternation) over what had occurred to him*" (Acts 3:10). A crowd gathered, and even though the man still clung firmly to Peter and John, Peter was quick to give Jesus the credit.

For a while, we may be crippled. We barely know how to beg for help. Others come along, and for a while we think they may be our salvation. We treasure their friendship, their caring, and their help. All the while, though it looks like them, it's really Jesus working in their hearts and our lives. They help us stand when we can't stand alone. They are Jesus with skin on. With their help, our ankle bones become stronger, and we learn to walk again.

This phrase "*leaping forth*" is so picturesque. Barely standing, then suddenly walking and even leaping forward, that former beggar praises God. How can a person walk and leap at the same time? I don't know, but I am determined to try. Won't you join me? May our legs walk forward into new life and our hearts leap forward in faith toward Christ. "*Behold, the Lord your God has set the land before you; go up and possess it, as the Lord, the God of your fathers, has said to you. Fear not, neither be dismayed*" (Deuteronomy 1:21).

Pages ago, we began to evaluate our hearts. Do we really believe all that we know about God? Will our devastating circumstances change truths we'd learned and rested in for years? As for me, I am once more able to take God at His Word and move steadfastly into my new land. It used to be called Widow, but I shall rename it Heartfelt.

My heart reels with feelings of loss right now and may do so for a long time, maybe even forever, but the God of all comfort continues to comfort me. Just read Isaiah 54:4–6 and discover how much He cares about widows:

Fear not, for you shall not be ashamed; neither be confounded and depressed, for you shall not be put to shame. For you shall forget the shame of your youth, and you shall not [seriously] remember the reproach of your widowhood any more. For your Maker is your Husband—the Lord of hosts is His name—and the Holy One of Israel is your Redeemer; the God of the whole earth He is called. For the Lord has called you like a woman forsaken, grieved in spirit, and heartsore—even a wife [wooed and won] in youth, when she is [later] refused and scorned, says your God.

My niece tells me that in playing cards, a "widow hand" is an extra hand of cards dealt face down whose value is not immediately known. For example, when you deal five cards up and two down, no one knows what the widow cards are. In fact, those very cards make the most difference in playing the hand you're dealt. Widowhood is the "extra card" God dealt me. Play it or pass it?

Attitude decides. This experience may become our most valuable possession if it makes us more like Christ. We only find out by walking through it, leaping forth in faith all the while.

Acts 3:16 says, *"[Jesus] has given the man this perfect soundness [of body]."* As we travel through pain, God heals our hearts. Just like in any heart surgery, scarring is part of the process. In spite of that scarring, our hearts function, keeping us alive and in the land of the living, not in the land of the half-dead from grief.

Verse 19 says, "*So repent (change your mind and purpose); turn around and return [to God], that your sins may be erased (blotted out, wiped clean), that times of refreshing (of recovering from the effects of heat, of reviving with fresh air) may come from the presence of the Lord.*" Doesn't this sound like recovery after sickness? I'm sure I made the right decision when I decided to trust God no matter what.

I wrote most of these chapters in longhand in my journals, without thought that they might see the light of day before I died and the family got their hands on them. I note my disjointed writing and missed letters, reread my writing and try to sneak the vowels into their proper places. An *N* and an *M* stand deformed. They join me in my disconnection and deformity.

Will I ever recover this side of heaven? We all know that answer: only by the grace of God.

I only mention this so you won't be afraid if it happens to you. It's just your way of going through. It is a picture of your life on paper.

Ron won't have to see me suffer, get sick, or die. He got frantic if I so much as sneezed. He wasn't one to visit hospitals. When the children were born it was all he could do to drop in for a half-hour visit.

Hospitals never bother me. I felt safe and comfortable there, always did. I had my tonsils out at age thirteen and never looked back. The only time I disliked a hospital was when Ron had his heart surgery, and that had nothing to do with Ron, the hospital, or me.

I ate for two when I was pregnant; now I must live for two. Then, I tried to pick foods to benefit both baby and me. Now Ron's earthly life is over, but I want his name to stand for something. I want to be a good steward of his death and to live

THE PREGNANT PAUSE OF GRIEF

my life well. This is a revelation to me, and I treasure it. When I think of Ron's death this way, it makes him live.

It is right and good to enjoy our families. When we make our new normal right and good, it is as much for them as it is for us.

Only God knows where our lives are going now. Should they be as they always were or change up? No one knows but Him, and He can help us face life with joy. We don't have to know how to deal with the holidays, because they aren't here yet.

Our family yearns for traditions that symbolize Ron's presence. This Christmas, I'm giving them copies of *The Big Red Chair*. I wrote all my love for God, Ron, and our family into that little children's book about grief, hoping it would comfort them.

Maybe we'll be afraid to mention Ron's name in case people cry. How could it spoil anything to remember the ones you loved, just because they now wait for you in a new place? Ron and his name always brought us joy before.

When Ron and I started dating, his family names and places seemed foreign to my uninitiated sixteen-year-old ears. I'd never heard of Lemonville, Rich Hill, or any of the other places the family talked about. Surely they'd made up those strange names! Years later, when we drove through those small communities, I saw them for myself.

Just like God says:

For now we are looking in a mirror that gives only a dim (blurred) reflection [of reality as in a riddle or enigma], but then [when perfection comes] we shall see in reality and face to face! Now I know in part (imperfectly), but then I shall know and understand fully and clearly, even in the same manner as I have been fully and clearly known and understood [by God] (1 Corinthians 13:12).

Just because we haven't heard it or seen it doesn't make it not so. Just because no one told us about Jesus doesn't make His truth less true. It does make us responsible to find out for ourselves. Unlike Thomas, we can believe without seeing if we've have started a personal relationship with Jesus Christ.

The Living Matter, and That Also Means Us

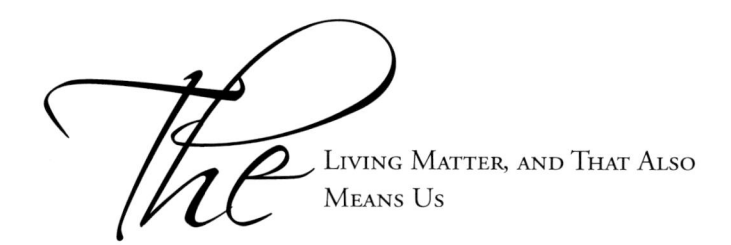

24

Okay means satisfactory, acceptable, all right, and even tolerable. Okay, then. I did not die when Ron died, even though at first it seemed so. It's okay to look after myself. Duty calls as it always has. I've always seen what was right and tried to do it. That explains why I offered to help a fellow student wipe up his vomit on the bus. It was the right thing to do. No one else did, and the bus driver's only solution was to hand the kid some paper towels.

I kept my mouth shut when it was often pointed out to me that the family home we bought was never really mine, that I did not belong there, and for that matter the things in it did not belong to me either. I never told Ron till we moved to this home, the first place I ever really thought of as mine.

'Why didn't you tell me that was going on?" he asked.

"Because I knew it would only cause trouble," I answered.

By the time I stood up for myself, everyone was so used to me rolling over and playing dead that it caused a major split in the family. The sleeping dog always arises to claim its territory.

People now say I'm courageous, but I am not—not brave, strong, or noble either. My strength only comes as I depend on Christ. I must go on, because the only other choice is stagnation.

When I saw the hit movie *The Help*, this line caught my attention: "Go find your life, Miss Skeeter." It brought me to tears because I'm now trying to find my life. For over fifty years, Ron was my life's chief purpose. I strived to maintain our relationship and be his best friend, lover, confidante, and, finally, caregiver.

Now, as I struggle to find fresh purpose, this one thing I know: "*He [God] Himself has said, I will not in any way fail you nor give you up nor leave you without support. [I will] not, [I will] not, [I will] not in any degree leave you helpless nor forsake nor let [you] down (relax My hold on you)! [Assuredly not!]*" (Hebrews 13:5).

If God says something once, it's worth listening to. If He says it twice, it's important. But three times? Sit up, pay attention, and stand in that promise!

Note: After writing this section about my need for purpose, I found this note from Ron taped to my desk. Surely I must have seen it before? But I don't remember it. Here it is:

Hello B. J. W.
Just a little note to let B. J. W. know
she is the love of my life for the rest of my life,
which should last for another sixty years or so.
Be ready, My Love, to tell the world of my God
and my love for you.
Love R. M. W.

THE PREGNANT PAUSE OF GRIEF

God answers prayer in the most astonishing ways. Once again, He reminded me to choose life. I first learned this when Ron and I were in the middle of wedding preparations for our son and his fiancée. That's when we got the doctor's diagnosis.

Ron didn't say a word until we got to the car. Then he took my hand and said, "We aren't telling anyone till after the wedding." I agreed to keep the secret, but I swallowed hard because anyone who knows me knows that I ask everyone to pray about everything. I kept my mouth shut all right, but my eyes wouldn't stop leaking.

Oh, I cried. I cried everywhere Ron wasn't and some places where he was. At church, I wept into his shoulder during worship. I sniffled through sermons and sobbed through prayer. Others knew only that our adult son was getting married. Since no one asked why I wallowed in tears, I presume they all surmised that I either hated my daughter-in-law-to-be or loved my son too much.

I wavered from joy to sorrow on a constant basis. Shower invitations cluttered the table while funeral thoughts swarmed my mind. I couldn't think straight. Tasks that my fingers previously flew through went unfinished. Half-baked projects littered the house. Meals were scattered at best and downright inedible at worst. It's not like I don't know how to cook, either. I come from a long line of prize-winning cooks, and I've also written several cookbooks.

I really let loose on my early morning walks. Practically galloping with stress, I'd pound my way around our little community, screaming my anguish at God. I demanded that He fix our life. I beseeched Him to restore Ron to health.

I despaired at losing Ron. "I've been married since I was eighteen, God. Our fortieth wedding anniversary is coming up.

Tell me, God, are we going to make it?" I just couldn't get a grip on the fact that our time together might soon end.

I'm ashamed to say I kept up this routine for weeks. Finally one morning, I ran out of words. My voice and my tears dried up. My mind went quiet too.

Into that deafening silence, God dropped these two words: "Choose life."

Choose life? What on earth did that mean? Would our circumstances change? Might Ron be healed? I rushed home to look those words up in my Bible.

"*This day I call the heavens and the earth as witnesses against you that I have set before you life and death, blessings and curses. Now choose life, so that you and your children may live*" (Deuteronomy 30:19, NIV). Oh.

During the last ten years of his life, Ron endured multiple bouts of chemotherapy, a hip replacement, a heart attack, and a triple bypass-valve repair. His life was in danger many times. Yes, I panicked through some of these events, but never to the extent of that first life-threatening news. We learned to live life in the present because Jesus gave us hope.

The Bible says that the God of our hope will "*so fill you with all joy and peace in believing [through the experience of your faith] that by the power of the Holy Spirit you may abound and be overflowing (bubbling over) with hope*" (Romans 15:13). To us, every day was a gift. We lived every day as though it was Christmas. We gave each other the gift of love every single day that we had together.

We celebrated every doctor's report, whether good or bad, because we learned that absolutely everything passed through God's hands before it got to us, and therefore it was life to us.

We chose to see chemotherapy as our friend. Because Ron and I knew Jesus as our personal Saviour, we expected to meet again in heaven someday. We counted on that because Jesus keeps His promises, and He promises us eternal life. So I must go on, because God, who gives life, expects us to choose life.

While the King James Version of Philippians 4:13 may be more familiar, "*I can do all things through Christ which strengtheneth me,*" I prefer the clarity of the Amplified Bible: "*I have strength for all things in Christ Who empowers me [I am ready for anything and equal to anything through Him Who infuses inner strength into me; I am self-sufficient in Christ's sufficiency].*"

Jesus, the Son of God, offers us real comfort and joy. "*The Lord God is my Strength, my personal bravery, and my invincible army; He makes my feet like hinds' feet and will make me to walk [not to stand still in terror, but to walk] and make [spiritual] progress upon my high places [of trouble, suffering, or responsibility]!*" (Habakkuk 3:19).

Ron spent ages waiting for me. I always needed one more trip to the bathroom or a tweak of my lipstick or even a run back into the house for the grocery list. Ron continues to wait for me now while God gets me ready for heaven.

We miss people all the time, even though they aren't dead. Distance is not a barometer of loneliness. I miss our children when they were six and ten and fifteen years old. I love who they are now, but I miss who they were just a little bit too. I miss the carefree little girl I was before abuse stole my childhood from me.

I Miss Ron

I miss; I miss our first tender kiss.
I miss the loving faces you sent me in all places.
I miss my heart on your sleeve, but not how I grieve.
Our love lasts forever, so, goodbye? It's never.

If we have arthritis, our knees ache on a rainy day while our joints swell to bursting. Our fingers twist and knot into peculiar positions. Some of us suffer from arthritis of the heart. Mine aches when I smell Ron's Old Spice cologne or his scent on the pillow. It twists when I remember his hugs, loving words, and endless supply of love for me. I'm glad I stored it up over the years so that I can pour out its memories all over again.

Why do we grieve? Why indeed? It's because grief is only another name for the love we shared. An absence of grief would mean we never cared. We've all known casual acquaintances who died, and while we were sorry about that, we didn't grieve for them much. We knew them, tolerated them, cared about them, but we never loved them with the deep, constant, enduring love we have for our own. We grieve deeply only for those people whom we love deeply. In an odd way, the torment of grief today is worth it, because it comes from knowing the depths of love.

Two Days Short of Knowing My Name

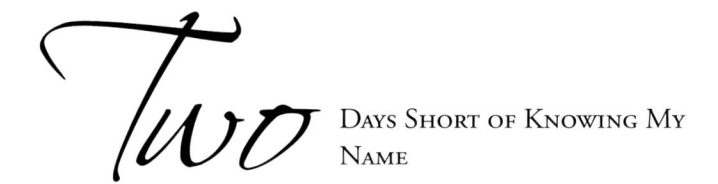

25

IN TWO DAYS IT WILL BE EXACTLY THREE MONTHS SINCE RON went to be with Jesus. I marvel that so much time passed in such a blur. Without this journal, I'd be hard pressed to remember any of it.

Only two more days now and I should be able to know my own name. I ask myself what that will feel like. I scarcely remember the sensation. Will it be like stepping into the sunshine after a long gloomy stay in a dungeon? Will it be like a bird on the wing for the first time or more like a toddler stepping, falling, catching a hand, being caught? I think so, because my name is no longer my name.

Three months ago I was Mrs. Ronald M. Wood. Now, according to the mail that arrives, I am suddenly just plain old Brenda Wood. With Ron, I was never plain anything. I was special, loved, and cherished. He thought me beautiful. He loved me "muchly."

"I love you muchly, Mrs. Wood," he'd say.

I used to be Mrs. Ronald M. Wood from the land of muchly loved. Now in the world's economy, I am barely a Ms. and certainly not a Mrs.

This strange new way of life skitters across my path every day as if surfacing for the very first time. I meet folks who don't know or just forgot, literally, that Ron died. I get mail with his name on it. Heart pangs attack me at certain scenes and happenings.

Take the mantel clock for instance. She's never been happy since Ron passed on. In all of Ron's seventy-six years, he heard that clock chime every day. He'd been responsible for her since his early teens. He wound her, kept her time straight, and knew how to make the chime and the hand point meld. She quit about a week before he died, and Ron directed me from his hospital bed so that I got her up and running again. He instructed me to push this and twizzle that. It took a bit of effort, but, finally, off she went, unashamed as I touched her innards. Bear in mind that I dusted her for nearly fifty years. Still, patting a gal on the shoulder is one thing. It's quite another to slide your hand into her nether regions.

But the moment Ron died, that chimer went into mourning. I've had no end of trouble with her. I wind her too tight or not tight enough. She strikes four, but the hands stay at eight. She stops because I forget to wind her. She even seems to need winding more often than before.

For me, she needs to run. She has to run. Like everything else around here, she's part of who we were as a couple. The longer Ron is away, the more I crave "sameness" in the form of everyday sanity.

THE PREGNANT PAUSE OF GRIEF

I can't stand to be with crazy folks, those who get upset over the smallest things. I want to scream when I hear women complain about their husbands' small foibles. I'm sorry for the times I complained about Ron's.

Ron loved a good joke. He'd tell one on the way into a room and one on the way out. He's likely told this one a few times: The trouble with some women is that they get all excited over nothing, and then they marry him.

I'd add this to his story: In my case, that nothing became everything.

Grief is like being a tree. One by one your limbs are yanked and pulled on until they separate from your body. It takes a long time to drag those limbs away, and even when they're gone, the open wounds remain. Oh yes, they heal in a funny fashion, but they leave behind discolouring and scarring and ooze.

The roots, though, are still in place, anchored in the depths of your memory. They are the memory of the couple you became when grafted together. To pull them out would mean to give up on living.

It seems too much to bear right now, but three months into this desert I discover, as you will too, that every day gets a little brighter. For me, it is possible now to walk past the men's clothing department without bursting into tears or remembering how I used to look for *that* colour of shirt or *that* length of jeans. It is possible to go to a Wendy's on my own and eat an Afi Burger and think about our happy conversations there. I entertain people in my home without apologizing for Ron's absence. I sleep through the night, dream of him, and wake grateful for the time we had together.

Am I happy about all that? No, not really, but it is reality and truth now. I am alone. In spite of my wonderful children and grandchildren, I am alone. Grieving is worse for a spouse because we've lost our other half. Children have their own families. They can mourn and be comforted there. They don't yet know the stinging loss of widowhood.

Anyway, I refuse to be a stalker. A stalker keeps trying to get close to a particular person. A grieving stalker wants her partner back because she doesn't feel whole without him. She makes a shrine of the family home. She desperately clings to her "missing piece." If we refuse to let our loved ones go, we become stalkers, chasing down a partner we no longer have.

Things are different now, but that does not mean that they're bad. It just means they're different. I led 4-H groups for years, and their motto applies now: "Learn to do by doing." We learn widowhood by doing. After all, behind every sweater is a lamb. Behind every child is a parent. Behind every answered prayer is a prayer. I'm learning to be a widow by being one.

Ron prayed faithfully for his wife and children every day. He repeatedly prayed for all the family members who had yet to meet Jesus. I expect he is still praying. He's finishing any of his unfinished earthly prayers in heaven!

> I can't get down upon my knees. They are a trifle bent.
> The surgery upon them has left them tired and bent.
> My heart yearns after Jesus; my legs they yearn that too.
> Everything about me craves relationship with You.
> So here I am a-standing, with heart now kneeling low
> I can't get down upon my knees as I did so long ago.

Oh, I haven't had surgery on my knees physically, only in my heart. The Lord took me down a peg or two in pride and a whole ladderful in attitude. He is God. He has the right to call His loved ones home to Himself. My right is to do what is right in God's eyes.

THE PREGNANT PAUSE OF GRIEF

Ron was anxious to go. He'd had enough pain and trouble. He just wanted Jesus. If I say I can't stand this journey through grief, I'm saying God's grace is not enough. Still, I hope both God and Ron forgive me when my passion does not equal their enthusiasm.

Ron left another little poem about God's garden of grace. Funny, I never heard him mention that phrase before, but now I find it in so many little scribbles.

> God's garden of grace is a wonderful place,
> Where we can look on my Saviour's face.
> Then wonders of love of men that He knows,
> The questions we'll ask and the answers are given.
> It'll all be done in God's wonderful grace.

It is not death to die if we know Jesus as our personal Saviour. Then death is simply moving into closer proximity to Him.

My granddaughter and I shared a leisurely trip to the library, followed by equally tranquil slices of pizza at a local shop. And it was all those things…until we opened the front door and remembered the eggs. Or rather, the eggs remembered us.

I'd thoughtlessly left a pan of eggs on the boil. Thankfully, only two of the five eggs made it to oblivion. The other three clung desperately to the base of the cooking pot, their little bottoms about the colour of God's good black planting soil.

You'd be surprised how far an egg can travel when it is heated beyond its blow-up point! Bits of shell, white, and entire yolks spread themselves a good twenty feet in diameter. Thankfully, we only used chicken eggs. Ostrich eggs would have travelled halfway to the Netherlands.

But listen to this! The yolks were mostly intact. The centres stayed in one piece! Yes, their edges were a little ragged, but they stayed strong and firm (very!).

I thought about the grieving process and how my centre is strong and firm because my centre is Jesus. "*Sing for joy, O heavens, and be joyful, O earth, and break forth into singing, O mountains! For the Lord has comforted His people and will have compassion upon His afflicted*" (Isaiah 49:13).

"*May your unfailing love be my comfort, according to your promise to your servant*" (Psalm 119:76, NIV). All that is left is the stinky egg smell, and that is not from God. The pain will pass. Why would I ever drag Ron back from his heavenly homecoming? Why desire to tie him to an earthly plain when he is in the heavenly? Some days I selfishly want to, but by the grace of God, I let go. And by doing so, I give Ron the freedom to enjoy his new life.

Stop Trying to Create Your Own Miracle

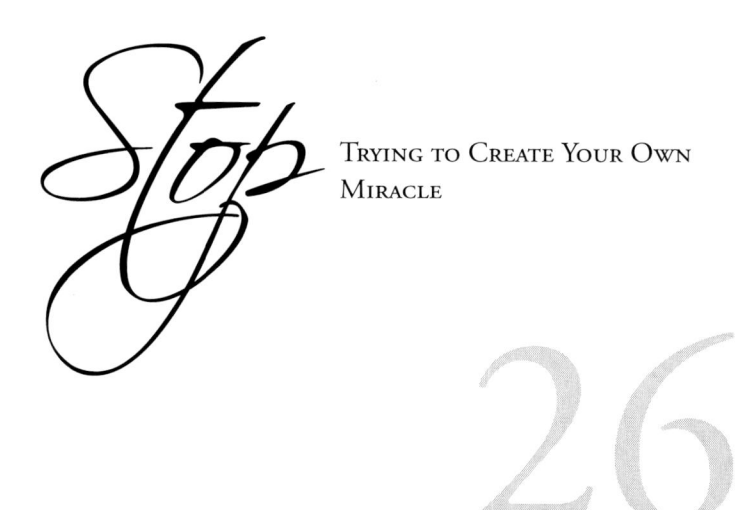

26

I've just watched that Christmas favourite *The Bishop's Wife* one more time. Cary Grant plays an angel who comes to earth in response to the bishop's (David Niven) request for help. When the help arrives in the form of an angel, the bishop refuses to believe that God sent him. In fact, he becomes quite jealous of the angel's presence. I realize we all get jealous once in a while, but of God's helpers and, therefore, of God Himself? That's scary.

Do we wish we'd been responsible for our big breakthrough, our own miracle? Do we treat God with little respect because we think we'd have done a better job, or do we want to take credit for what happened to us? Are we proud of ourselves because we think it was all our idea?

As I look back on my journals I find many blessings from God. Perhaps I took them as my own when they happened. I hope not.

For instance, on the spur of the moment last December 18, we got tickets to our local restaurant for their special Christmas dinner event. Ron was well enough to go. I remember thinking it was expensive at the time, but now I cherish the time we had there.

The year before that, someone gave us their New Year's Eve tickets. We'd stopped buying event tickets long before that, simply because we didn't know how Ron would be feeling on any given day. So we had a lovely evening with friends because of the kindness of others.

I wonder now if Ron made himself go to events when they turned up like this because he knew I might like them or because he wanted us to have one more good memory. That New Year's party was definitely special. It was our last evening out and our last public dance. The memory clings to my heart like glue. I sense his arms around me and his dipping me in the waltzes like he always did.

I had a guy who did his best no matter what. No matter the pain, the hardship, or the sorrow, Ron always found a good place in the midst of it. So how would Ron look at this situation, and what would he do to find the good place?

He'd go out with people and smile through hurt. He'd continue to love me from afar, enjoy his children and grandchildren. He might not write a book for the grieving little ones, but he would tell them what a great gal I was, how much he loved me, and how much I loved them. He'd keep my memory alive with funny stories of our times together and gaze at my picture like he used to gaze at me when he thought I wasn't looking.

THE PREGNANT PAUSE OF GRIEF

When I consider Ron's failing health and the gift of extra time both he and God gave to me, how can I negate them now? How can I discount either one? I am loved.

I'm not saying that I have this all together, that I have it made. But I am well on my way, reaching out for Christ, who has so wondrously reached out for me. Friends, don't get me wrong: By no means do I count myself an expert in all of this, but I've got my eye on the goal, where God is beckoning us onward—to Jesus. I'm off and running, and I'm not turning back (Philippians 3:12–14, MSG).

The Bible says our joy can be full (1 John 1:4) and that the joy of the Lord is our strength (Nehemiah 8:10).

Like me, you probably skip over the parts of Ecclesiastes 3:1–14 you don't like.

There is an appointed time for everything. And there is a time for every event under heaven—A time to give birth and a time to die; A time to plant and a time to uproot what is planted. A time to kill and a time to heal; A time to tear down and a time to build up. A time to weep and a time to laugh; A time to mourn and a time to dance. A time to throw stones and a time to gather stones; A time to embrace and a time to shun embracing. A time to search and a time to give up as lost; A time to keep and a time to throw away. A time to tear apart and a time to sew together; A time to be silent and a time to speak. A time to love and a time to hate; A time for war and a time for peace (Ecclesiastes 3:1–8, NASB).

Everything on earth has its own time and its own season. Of course, we'd all agree to this. Not too personal yet, right?

There is a time for both birth and death. Yes, we like this, especially if we get the birth part and the death is someone else's.

Planting and reaping? I come from a farm. I know this stuff.

Isn't it interesting that healing and building come after killing and destroying? That confirms the thought that all things happen for our good.

Meanwhile, the moment we get tired in the waiting, God's Spirit is right alongside helping us along. If we don't know how or what to pray, it doesn't matter. He does our praying in and for us, making prayer out of our wordless sighs, our aching groans. He knows us far better than we know ourselves, knows our pregnant condition, and keeps us present before God. That's why we can be so sure that every detail in our lives of love for God is worked into something good (Romans 8:28, MSG).

First we have crying and weeping, but laughing and dancing follow. Perhaps throwing stones and gathering stones refer to the anger some of us have as part of the grieving process?

I love the embracing part, but for each of us, at some point, parting follows. I found Ron, or maybe he found me. It was wonderful, but again, losing is part of life.

God gave me Ron to keep for almost fifty years, and then God asked me to give him back. How can I refuse the request of God? I can cling to what used to be our life or let God have His way and lean forward into our someday, the day I will meet Ron once more, in God's garden.

So now we are on one of my favourite subjects, sewing. Jesus liked it too! "*No one cuts up a fine silk scarf to patch old work clothes; you want fabrics that match*" (Luke 5:36, MSG).

Here we are in this new place. We can't continue to patch our old life into the new one. It's time to find out who we are and to make decisions with God's help. This brings us closer to God and what He wants for us. Sometimes we'll spend a whole half day without tears. We'll find a cherished memory soothing. We'll give kindness to others experiencing the same pain.

I listen to God more, and I lean on Him for the words I need to say. This book is so much of God and so little of me. I'd like to keep my life on that track.

I love greatly because I am greatly loved. The war in my mind settles as I work on this book. I know who I am again. I always was a child of God, and so I find myself again. To the world I may no longer be Mrs. Ronald M. Wood, but in my heart I know who I am. *"My beloved is mine and I am his"* (Song of Songs 2:16, NIV).

And look at you! You're wearing the same name tag as me, "Beloved Child of God"! In His eyes we are

- B being
- E eternally
- L loved
- O overwhelmingly
- V valued and
- E endlessly
- D dear!

And Ecclesiastes goes on…

What do we gain by all our hard work? God sometimes demands difficult things from us, yet God also makes everything happen at the right time. None of us ever fully understands. He puts questions in our minds about the past and the future.

I surely questioned God, but in searching for the answers I found Him all over again. I come to this conclusion: We are to enjoy our lives, just like it says in John 10:10, because God's gift to us is peace and contentment in Him. "*The thief comes only in order to steal and kill and destroy. I came that they may have and enjoy life, and have it in abundance (to the full, till it overflows).*"

The thief thought to destroy our lives, but instead, in spite of the circumstances, we found God to be deeper and purer, more comforting than ever. We found ourselves where we did not want to be, but even Jesus had to do that. John 4:4 says it was necessary for Jesus to go through Samaria.

Were Ron and I tired of our Samaria? You bet. Did we every wonder why we were still in it? You bet. Then one day our neighbour told us she had cancer.

"I'm okay with it, Ron. I've seen you stand through all these things. I know I can do it too."

She started coming to church, and someday, I pray, she'll find Jesus for herself.

Jews in New Testament times travelling from Judea to Galilee or vice versa would cross over the Jordan River, avoid Samaria by going through Transjordan, and cross back over the river again once they reached their destination. Nobody wanted to be in Samaria.

The Bible says that Jesus was there by necessity. Why did he bother? He could have avoided it. I mean, He was Jesus, after all! It wasn't a safe place for a Jew to be, yet he found rest and refreshment there (John 4:6–8). He enjoyed conversation (4:7) and confrontation (4:9) and had a chance to witness (4:10–24).

As a result a woman chose to believe in Christ (4:25–26). She left to tell others about Jesus (4:29), and they also believed (4:41).

THE PREGNANT PAUSE OF GRIEF

If we balk, whine, complain, and moan about the hardships and difficulties of our less-than-safe place, I doubt our neighbours will be looking for Jesus. I'm grateful that Jesus left a blueprint of how to get through Samaria.

And finally, that last little bit of Ecclesiastes chapter 1? Everything God has done will last forever; nothing He does can ever be changed. God has done all this so that we will worship Him. We'll see our loved ones again. God says so.

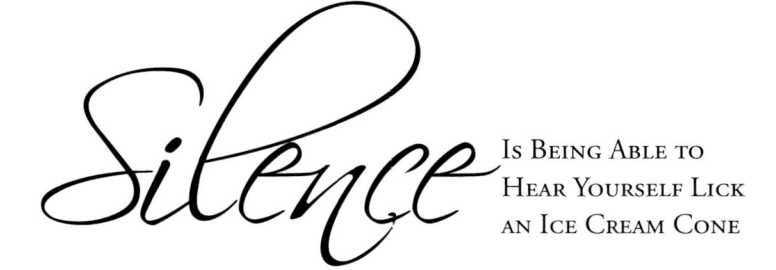

Silence Is Being Able to Hear Yourself Lick an Ice Cream Cone

27

Purpose

The purpose wasn't clear back then. It seemed a senseless act.
Many blamed our Father God, and that's the simple fact.
And then folks started saying it was for us to choose the Lord
And deeply, in the simplest sense, into our life He poured.
But oh, dear ones, can you see it now, the truth you get to tell?
For God makes plans for all to hear. Go tell the story well.

God may close a door, but He always opens a window. If we keep looking at closed doors, we never find the windows.

> When the righteous cry for help, the Lord hears, and delivers them out of all their distress and troubles. The Lord is close to those who are of a broken heart and saves such as are crushed with sorrow for sin and are humbly and

thoroughly penitent. Many evils confront the [consistently] righteous, but the Lord delivers him out of them all (Psalm 34:17–19).

The day we celebrated Ron's life, we all talked about what a great guy he is (sorry; sometimes I still talk present tense). We shared memories and ate birthday cake. Yes, you heard right. I ordered ten birthday cakes for Ron's special day. They were inscribed with the words "Welcome Home." After all, we were celebrating his homecoming, the day he went to be with Jesus.

Anyway, Ron thoroughly disliked "funeral" food. Musty tuna salad with mayo, ham chopped beyond recognition, egg salad without onion, and phoney turkey made him leery. He'd say, "There's never a decent roast beef sandwich in the lot." You can see why we haunted the nearest Wendy's restaurant after these occasions. That was our usual "funeral" day.

But after Ron's cake and coffee, others probably discussed how awful the food was, how great the music, and how maudlin the family speeches. However, I drove home in lonely silence to a lonely home…only to find the Holy Spirit waiting there for me. I am alone, but not lonely, because God lives in my house. Ron left me in good hands. "*GOD's loyal love couldn't have run out, his merciful love couldn't have dried up. They're created new every morning. How great your faithfulness! I'm sticking with GOD (I say it over and over). He's all I've got left*" (Lamentations 3:22–23, MSG).

Thankfully, I've learned to stick with God's advice. You'd be surprised at the advice you get.

"Get out of the house." I heard this from three separate people in three different countries. I chose not to listen. It felt good to cry, so I did. Finally, God reminded me that I am known for my common sense. So I thought I'd better get some.

THE PREGNANT PAUSE OF GRIEF

Someone reminded me that even in laughter the heart may ache. Then I read that I should choose which side of the ache to stand on. (Oh, who said that? Let me think—It was me! At the last minute I'd added those scribbled words to my message at Ron's going-home-to-Jesus party.

I've decided to stand on the side of joy for Ron's sake and for mine. I don't have to feel happy to put a smile on my face. God is faithful and true no matter what. I trust God to tell me what to do. My needs are provided for in a myriad of ways that would take a book all on their own. I continue to follow God's advice. Choose life.

Oh, and did I tell you? Just after I posted Ron's note about being ready "to tell the world of my God and my love for you" I got a call for a speaking engagement. God is working His plan. "Fresh…your grief is still so fresh," people say. Because you might also need refreshing, the information follows.

"*He makes me lie down in [fresh, tender] green pastures*" (Psalm 23:2). As a kid, I lay in fresh pastures at our farm, inhaling the intoxicating blooms of alfalfa and clover. The bed of green cushioned and comforted me. I could see the blue of the heavens above. Today God offers cushioning and comfort when we fix our eyes on Him. This peace happens, not because we are worth it, but because it is God's nature to offer it.

"*Sustain me with raisins, refresh me with apples, for I am sick with love*" (Song of Solomon 2:5). I guess you can say that I am sick with love, missing my Honey, but at least proper eating, exercise, and several glasses of water daily do make a difference in my physical state. A ton of books insist you can change a habit in twenty-one days. Stop smoking, lose weight, and stop biting your nails. Don't you believe it. Three months have not made me prefer living without Ron, and I doubt three years will either. I prefer Ron here, but that's not possible, so I must move on.

"*Repent, then, and turn to God, so that your sins may be wiped out, that times of refreshing may come from the Lord*" (Acts 3:19, NIV). We knew this, right? But a reminder didn't hurt me and likely won't bother you any.

At first I felt guilty. How could I be having fun without Ron? Then I remembered how much he enjoyed life, and I thought about what another friend told me. "Take care of yourself, Brenda. Ron would want you to do that." And he would. "*Weeping may endure for a night, but joy cometh in the morning*" (Psalm 30:5, KJV).

Ron's death affects so much of my life. I've been on the speaking circuit for years, but now Ron isn't here to mark out my driving trail. Computer mapping and I are now best friends. I practice my speeches in an empty room. Two writing awards came in the mail yesterday, but I can't share them with him.

Our mail file at church now says "RBrenda Wood." The new slip of paper doesn't quite cover his name. It stands as a silent reminder that Ron used to be there but is no longer. No one noticed but me.

We need to pray that we will continue to give strong testimony, that our emotions will behave themselves and stay under the rule of the Holy Spirit. Just in these short few months, others have lost their spouses. Now it is my turn to help them. As the Bible says,

He comes alongside us when we go through hard times, and before you know it, he brings us alongside someone else who is going through hard times so that we can be there for that person just as God was there for us. We have plenty of hard times that come from following the Messiah, but no more so than the good times of his healing comfort—we get a full measure of that, too (2 Corinthians 1:4–5, MSG).

THE PREGNANT PAUSE OF GRIEF

LEARNING THE LANGUAGE OF WIDOW

We started out all brave and sure of the path we were to take.
But then it looked too difficult. Our strength we had to fake.
The people strange, the rules unclear,
we stumbled on some more.
We couldn't seem to fit in, so why the open door?
The language was all funny. The words so hard to say.
We couldn't get our tongue around the topic of the day.
The pain was all a blur of words, the *widow* word just bad.
We tried another version and it was just as sad.
We struggled on, until we saw we'd found the perfect place.
We were on the common pathway.
We'd joined the widow race.
So though we speak it clearly now, we still remember when
That new life was all weird to us, so we help others,
when we can.

"Death is a big relief to them." This comment shocked me at first, but as I pondered it, I sensed its truth. Of course, Ron didn't want to leave us, but his heart turned toward heaven long before he moved there.

Little by little, the foods Ron loved became less important to him. Our hamburger king (who would eat it three times a day if possible) lost his taste for Wendy's and even homemade meatloaf. I bought treats to tempt his appetite, but after one nibble, the rest of the goodie would sit abandoned.

He chided me for running around and cleaning, doing dishes and so on. "Just sit down and be quiet with me," he'd say. "You can do that stuff later." So I did. Ron's clock was set on heaven's time, while I continued on Eastern Standard. Eventually he didn't even want to hear his beloved country music. The closer he got to God, the less he craved earth's pleasures. He wasn't able to do the things he used to do, but he enjoyed the things he could still do, like praying.

Less time for earth's pleasures gave him more time for fellowship with God, and the more time he spent with God, the more he looked forward to being with Him.

What if we were all craving fellowship with God long before He called us home? More time with God would mean less time to binge eat or drink or dope up, less time in the mall buying stuff we don't need, and less time in unforgiveness. And more time with God would get us ready for the time when we will be with Him in a brand new way.

Have you ever been just *so* close to your goal and then missed the mark by *this* much? And that meant you had to start all over again? When I fell, I had to get up and try those blessed stairs one more time. There was no other way but up. "*But let endurance and steadfastness and patience have full play and do a thorough work, so that you may be [people] perfectly and fully developed [with no defects], lacking in nothing*" (James 1:4).

Emotions run deep, drain my being, and knot my stomach. Pick one. Just pick one. You have them, and so do I. I'd like to tackle one at a time, if they would be so gracious as to show up that way. Ha!

Anger, sadness, resentment, denial, rage, loneliness, jealousy, inadequacy, rejection, confusion, helplessness, guilt, anxiety, disappointment, pain, dread, bitterness, fear, envy, depression, loss, anguish, dismay, sorrow, betrayal, abandonment, apathy, distrust, and lack of control beseige me.

And crying attends every one. Yesterday in the midst of an outburst, my friend ignored my tears and just asked this question: "Does that just happen? Like out of nowhere?"

And I tell her what I've told you so many times in this book. "Yes. Yes!" Life is not the way it's supposed to be. It is the way it is. The way we cope with it makes the difference. I thought of the doubled-over lady in Luke 13:11. It's hard to make spiritual progress when all you see is your own dirty feet. But Jesus called her to healing. He did the straightening. All she had to do was look up.

I'm only in the first trimester of grief. Parts of me are still bent out of shape, but at least I know the cure. Look up.

When our hearts are heavy with sadness, others don't always feel the same depth of pain. Friends and family members jolly us along. Our sadness drags them down. All we want is to be alone, cry healing tears, treasure a little peace and quiet, and ponder what to do under the circumstances. Instead we may hear words like this: "Get over it! Your husband has been dead for two months already. Get a life. Lighten up. Your constant crying is depressing."

"For there they who led us captive required of us a song with words, and our tormentors and they who wasted us required of us mirth, saying, Sing us one of the songs of Zion" (Psalm 137:3). Where can we go in the midst of our suffering when friends don't understand? Only one place offers healing in every situation. *"This is my comfort and consolation in my affliction: that Your word has revived me and given me life"* (Psalm 119:50).

Of course the time will come when we are able to enjoy life again and face the future in the midst of our new circumstances, but until then? Let's cling to the promise in Psalm 138:7. Though we walk in the midst of trouble, God will revive us! *"They who sow in tears shall reap in joy and singing"* (Psalm 126:5).

"Who dares despise the day of small things...?" (Zechariah 4:10, NIV).

"What, then, shall we say in response to these things? If God is for us, who can be against us?" (Romans 8:31, NIV).

From Ron's Point of View

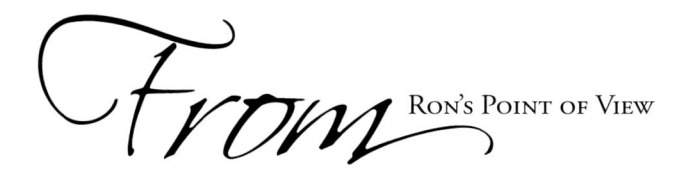

28

PART ONE: THE EARLY DAYS

I HAD A REPUTATION FOR HEAVY DRINKING, RUNNING THE ROADS and partying. The neighbourhood "bad" boy, I dropped out of school at fourteen and went to work with Dad on the farm. I also hired out to other odd jobs on occasion. It was what kids did then. A girl stayed home for Mom and a guy for Dad. I got my high school entrance, and that was all a kid needed, especially if you had a strong back, like I did.

In 1959, I met the love of my life, but she had plans for law school and was ten years younger than me. Still, we married in 1963 when I was the ripe old age of twenty-eight and she was eighteen. We farmed a bit, and I worked out some and drove tractor-trailer a bit. We never had much money, but we were so happy. Judith and Charles liked nothing better than to go on a trip with me in that old truck. They still swoon at the whiff of burning diesel fuel, but the truck kept me away too much. Brenda and the children missed me a lot.

I tried other jobs, even factory work. Not so keen on that one. When I got hired as a mechanic's apprentice, it only encouraged my love of John Deere equipment. I earned my license in farm machinery, then propane. Along the way I picked up some welding skills. Dozens of other tickets (licenses) followed.

Everyone we knew sent their kids to Sunday school to get a few minutes of peace and quiet. We did that for a long time, but one day Brenda asked Jesus into her life. It was all foreign to me, but things got better at home.

Over the next little while, both children asked Jesus into their lives too. I was the only holdout. I remember telling Brenda that I was working on getting good enough to get saved. The truth is that I couldn't stand it much longer. I got tired of the three of them talking about problems and then asking God for help. God always helped them too. I wanted what they had.

Finally one day, I got it. Jesus loved me just the way I was. Nothing I did would make Him love me more. He really did die on the cross, and He rose from the dead just for me. I asked him to forgive my sins, come into my life, and He did, just like that. We all began to change and grow as we learned more about God.

Our lifestyle of weekend parties dwindled. We discovered we'd rather be together as a family. Even when our teenagers started dating, Brenda and I just wanted to be together. After all, we barely got to do that during the week.

I wasn't surprised when the boss told me that we'd be going to a four-day workweek. Business was poor, and a slow winter season lay ahead. I was fifty-five, the economy was in a slump, and everyone seemed to want to tell me stories about older men losing their jobs. I went home and told my wife. I reminded her that God was faithful and that He never lets us down. I think I convinced her, but I was having a hard time convincing myself.

Monday provided less work than Friday. My day off was supposed to be Wednesday, but I left by noon. I find it harder to pretend to be busy than to actually be busy. I faced a future of three days' pay for the week. It would never cover our living expenses.

On the way home, I stopped to buy gas. I had a lawn mower in the back that I'd been trying to sell for at least three months. The stranger at the next gas pump bought it off the back of my truck! As I drove on, a company name came to me. I'd never tried there for a job, but they might have jobs for truck drivers. I had my AZ (tractor-trailer permit) license, and even though I'd rather do mechanical work, I felt I could go back to the trucks. The manager told me to come right over.

I made up a resume and decided to visit a friend who lived in the area. His road was closed, and I had to drive past another repair shop, so I stopped in and asked about a job. They needed a man one day a week! By the time I got home, the first company had called and wanted me to start, not as a truck driver but as plant manager! That one day all the skill I'd been learning for years came together in one.

God had more in mind that just a job. After only a few weeks, psoriasis, caused by grease cleansers, disappeared from my hands. Blood clots in my feet, from constant standing on cement floors, disappeared because now I walk all day. And every time I tell this story, both my listeners and I get a fresh glimpse of God's great faithfulness. "*The LORD's lovingkindnesses indeed never cease, For His compassions never fail. They are new every morning; Great is Your faithfulness*" (Lamentations 3:22–23, NASB).

Part Two: Gentleman's Agreement

I lay on the hospital stretcher, trying to remain calm. A chain had snapped loose from a truck and smashed into my face. The doctor, my wife, and the pastor had all been in to see me, but now I was alone because everyone thought I was in the operating room. Not so. A bad highway accident postponed my appointment with the surgeons.

The surgery would leave my teeth wired together for a minimum of six weeks while my jaw, broken in ten places, would hopefully heal. I might be disfigured. Infection was a distinct risk. For six weeks, I'd be on liquids only.

I knew and trusted the Lord. I knew He'd care for us, but this was a hard thing. Brenda had just had her second cancer surgery, and both our children had been ill. I'd be an added burden.

Finally, eleven hours after the accident, we got started. I had an unknown allergy to Demerol. It took a while to stabilize me. Then the doctors struggled with the placement of my jaw bones.

When you're alone, I mean *really* alone, with no loved ones to hold your hand, where do you turn? Thankfully, I knew enough to turn to God. "*Surely God is my salvation; I will trust and not be afraid. The Lord, the Lord himself, is my strength and my defense; he has become my salvation*" (Isaiah 12:2, NIV).

Almost six hours later, jaw screwed together, I was wheeled back to my room. I found myself in the very place I hated, a hospital. On top of that, I was sicker than anyone I'd ever seen. I had tubes coming out of places all over my body.

I thought of the times I should have stayed at the bedside of friends and, yes, even family. I just couldn't make myself do it. Isn't it amazing how God takes your fears and plunks you right down in the middle of them?

Since I couldn't run, I did the next best thing. I began to pray. As I lifted up my hand to praise God, to my astonishment I felt a squeeze on my hand. I knew it was the Lord. There was no one else there. I was raised to trust a man by his handshake. All my life I've made lots of purchases and sales on the strength of that. There was no mistaking the promise in this one. The Lord confirmed in my heart what I knew in my head. He was with me. The memory of that handshake sustained me through the trying times ahead. "*I am holding you by your right hand—I, the Lord your God—and I say to you, Don't be afraid; I am here to help you*" (Isaiah 41:13, TLB).

Later, the doctors confirmed that if I'd been a smoker or a drinker, I'd have bled to death on the way to the hospital. The chain hit my jaw and not my throat, so I didn't suffocate. My neck didn't break because my head was thrown against a truck. The lump from that blow was a small price to pay. My upper denture, thirty-six years old and obviously made by a master craftsman, hadn't broken, so the surgeon was able to mould my broken bones around it. My only scar is the small incision necessary for that screw.

While the Lord held my hand, our church came alongside. A friend refused to get me what he called wimpy flowers. He had an arrangement delivered in a John Deere model tractor and wagon. I worked for John Deere for twenty-plus years, and I still get teased about having green blood.

People did chores and delivered meals. They kept me company when Brenda was at work. Less than a month later, I was back at work, jaw still wired, drinking liquid everything. Brenda even figured out how to puree pizza! I thank God for saving my life during that traumatic time. Today, I am exactly where God wants me to be because He still holds my hand.

Part Three: Wait on the Lord
(Ron gave this message at our church about eighteen months before he died.)

As most of you know, I've had a few issues with my health over the years. In 1991, just after Brenda's first cancer surgery, an accident at work left me with a jaw broken in ten places.

Then in 1992, Brenda had her second cancer surgery and I broke my back at work. I developed diabetes then. I had a heart attack a few years ago and then had my left hip replaced. I've had chronic lymphatic leukemia since 2001, and that meant lots of chemotherapy.

Through all this, no one listened when I complained about pains around my middle. The doctor said it was likely heartburn or indigestion, so we believed him. I had lots of bad nights when I had to sit up. I often couldn't breathe, especially when I was taking chemotherapy treatments. My arms ached all the time. I had no energy. We blamed it on the chemotherapy.

I found that I couldn't even walk short distances, and again we blamed it on the chemotherapy and the cancer. My cancer doctor finally sent me to the hospital emergency room for heart tests.

The doctor on call immediately put me on beta blockers, baby aspirin, and nitro patches. Before we even left the hospital, he found me a heart specialist. In no time, that doctor diagnosed blockages in my heart and booked an angiogram for me.

Because my last chemotherapy worked so well, my white cells went down to normal. My red cells were too low, but my first blood transfusion helped me get some

THE PREGNANT PAUSE OF GRIEF

energy back. All in all, we celebrated our 46th wedding anniversary with me feeling pretty good.

The angiogram on March 9th showed an enlarged heart with a 90 to 100 percent blockage. I also had damage on the bottom of my heart. Suddenly I was on the urgent list for emergency bypass surgery. They said, "Go home and take it easy till we call you!"

We saw God do miracles every single day. For example, the cancer doctor's permission for me to have surgery got to the heart doctor's office before they knew I was going to be their patient. It didn't hurt that Brenda put me on every prayer list there was. I got emails from all around the world. As usual, church friends brought food, sent cards, and supported us in every way.

I met my wonderful surgeon, a little Egyptian guy. We spotted him right off as a Christian. His office was full of paintings and statues with only one theme. A patient is on an operating table, the surgeon is operating, and Jesus stands behind him, guiding his hands. We knew we were in the right place. We relaxed and did exactly what all the medical staff said to do. "Go home and wait till we call you."

March 29, I awoke in the night with terrible chest pain. Here's just a small note of advice for you. Always call 911 and the ambulance! They know how to diagnose and treat your problems. Right off they gave me three chewable baby aspirins and a nitro spray treatment. I ended up going to hospital by ambulance. They kept me there on oxygen, and I was glad to stay. Hospital heart patients get fast-tracked to surgery.

They moved me to another hospital on April 2nd, and I was scheduled for a triple bypass and a valve repair on the 3rd of April. I was in the operating room by 7 a.m. on April 3rd for almost six hours. I have a scar the full length of my chest. By half past two, Brenda and our daughter were allowed in. Brenda said there were so many tubes in my chest that she couldn't have put her two hands around them all.

I got out of the intensive care unit by noon the next day. I expect prayer played a big part. I was five hours ahead of schedule. The staff taught me how to get out of bed without too much pain and how to climb stairs easier, and so on. By the third day, they pulled all the chest wires out. That was an experience because they were each about fourteen inches long. By Thursday we were on our way home!

You know, we think little children don't know what is going on, but we are wrong. Our granddaughter, only two at the time, came to visit and right away covered me with my John Deere blanket and got me a pillow for behind my back.

Little by little, I got better and gradually recovered my strength. One of my best experiences was that two days after surgery, I said to Brenda—"I *can breath*!"

She said, "What are you talking about?"

"I can breathe—I can really take a deep breath and breathe! I haven't done that for years," and I grinned.

Right now I'm really healthy. We see God's hand in our lives every day. We experience miracles regularly. My cancer is under control, and every day is a blessing. We know that what comes to us always first passes through God's hands. And we can face it all, because

He's going through every bit of it with us. "*God made my life complete when I placed all the pieces before him*" (2 Samuel 22:21, MSG).

People wonder why I'm so fond of eagles. Well, when my back was broken and I couldn't walk, and when I had a broken jaw and I couldn't talk properly, I found these verses in my Bible:

Have you not known? Have you not heard? The everlasting God, the Lord, the Creator of the ends of the earth, does not faint or grow weary; there is no searching of His understanding. He gives power to the faint and weary, and to him who has no might He increases strength [causing it to multiply and making it to abound]. Even youths shall faint and be weary, and [selected] young men shall feebly stumble and fall exhausted; But those who wait for the Lord [who expect, look for, and hope in Him] shall change and renew their strength and power; they shall lift their wings and mount up [close to God] as eagles [mount up to the sun]; they shall run and not be weary, they shall walk and not faint or become tired (Isaiah 40:28–31).

That Was Then...This Is Now

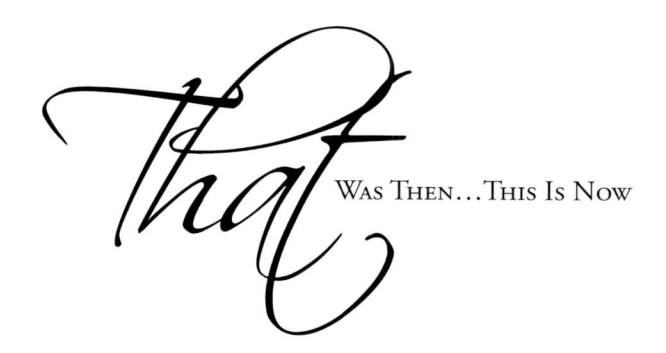

29

SIX WEEKS AFTER RON'S DEATH
We laughed and ate and shared our scribbles at one of the best Writers' Nest meetings ever. It left me with a peculiar, unrecognized feeling. Finally it came to me. The feeling was joy! I was having a wonderful time!

At first I felt guilty. How could I be having fun without Ron? Then I remembered how much my Ron enjoyed life. *"Weeping may endure for a night, but joy comes in the morning"* (Psalm 30:5).

Yesterday the first copies of my first children's book, *The Big Red Chair*, arrived at my door. It is a happy, funny, sad love story about life and death. I wrote it for our smaller grandchildren who don't understand what happened to their Afi. I expect lots of other little ones feel the same. We often unknowingly and unfairly lock them out of our grief.

THREE MONTHS LATER
For the past few years, I've been accused of doing something I did not do, and it has been hard to just be quiet and say nothing. The unfairness of the thing bothered Ron terribly, and he was angry on my account.

God expects us to forgive. When Ron was dying, I asked him if he had been able to forgive, and though he was barely able to talk by then, he uttered out a firm "Yep!" I told him that I too had forgiven the people involved. We found joint peace together. Forgiveness brings peace, comfort and relief.

FOUR MONTHS LATER
Eating well? How could I not be eating well? Friends stocked my freezer, and I choose from a restaurant-like menu. Shall I eat lasagna, potato soup, or chicken this day? Or should I investigate spaghetti, pork chops, and more? I pridefully refused these gifts when they were first offered. Someone else needs it more, I declared. All of that might be true, but on a teary day like today, those meals feed my body, mind, soul, and spirit. I remember each giver with thanks and great appreciation for their kindnesses to me and vow to be grateful…just because I can. "*I thank my God in all my remembrance of you*" (Philippians 1:3).

FIVE MONTHS LATER
The first copies of *Meeting Myself: Snippets from a Binging and Bulging Mind* arrived today.

And all I could think was "I wish Ron was here to share this with me." And I cried.

What's that? Didn't want to read my own new book? Cared not to see the words in actual print?

No. Read it one hundred times while writing, editing, and preparing for the book launch.

I worked myself into a frenzy of grief from 2:00 when it arrived till 7:20 p.m. and ate to "comfort" my heart. Note: your drug of choice cannot make your heart happy.

Anyway, finally at 7:20 common sense reared its pretty little head once more—and because the ice cream was all gone, I opened to the dedication page. "For Ron, who walked with me every step of the way."

And the thought came to me that Ron knew that his job was done here. He'd seen me safely into healing and completeness. He knew that bulimia and its related attacks had no more power over me. He knew I had the strength to carry on because I'd found the Christ, the truth of all life.

Six Months Later

Because of a water tank episode, the flooring in my house is being replaced. That sounds lovely, doesn't it? Who wouldn't want to have new flooring, new desk, new colours, even a new wallpaper border? Me, that's who.

I burst into tears in the store because nothing will look like it did when Ron was here. The saleslady cried too. She just lost her mom, and so we blubbered together.

Now china cabinet contents explode onto every flat surface. The china cabinet itself sits in front of the living room window. I can't even see the TV. The chairs are too cluttered to sit on. I have one tiny walking path through the house, which I dare not use without flashlight in hand.

My house looks as bad as I feel. But there is that one little path through and that one glimmer of hope and light and that one hand to hold. So Christ and I move through together toward healed house and healed heart.

SEVEN MONTHS AFTER RON'S DEATH
This month holds both our 49th wedding anniversary and Ron's birthday. We always celebrated the two special days with gusto. I'm concentrating on some of those sweet memories now. I hope you are celebrating something special with your loved ones today. Make every day worthwhile. You never know…It might be the last one you have together. *"Woe is me for my hurt! My wound is grievous; but I said, Truly this is a grief, and I must bear it"* (Jeremiah 10:19, *KJV*).

EIGHT MONTHS LATER
I'm editing *The Pregnant Pause of Grief*. It rips at my heart just as much as it did when I first wrote it. Does grief ever go away? I don't think so. Does it become a little less raw? Maybe, but I don't know that yet. Do hearts ache because they are full of love and have nowhere to put it?

Does God still comfort and console? Of course He does, or else He wouldn't be God.

In spite of that, I wallow in avoidance, tears, and self-pity. I am overtired. When I can't write, I know I am not right within myself. Food and I continue to be warring friends. I tell myself that it is okay to abuse food. After all, it abused me for years! I could go on, but why bore you unmercifully…I need a good old-fashioned dose of common sense.

As St Augustine said, "Drunkenness is far from me. Thou wilt grant in thy mercy that it never approach me. But gluttony sometimes steals upon thy servant."

No Longer

An eating binge, a total fast;
Bad habits, Lord, that seem to last.
Too much today, tomorrow naught.
Oh Lord, the cookies that I've bought
For "visitors" have disappeared…
And it is just as I had feared.
My gluttony destroyed the box.
I lied about them like a fox.
My gluttony, Lord, is destroying me.
Help me to fight former slavery.
You promised that in Christ, I'm free.
Oh, Lord, keep on reminding me…
That you have made me new and clean.
I'm now no longer what I've been.
(Based on Romans 6:11–14)

Nine Months Later

Great news! Common sense just showed up and, might I say, not a minute too soon!

I've been in a "freeze heave" situation. The frost of grief left a lump in my path. As you know from earlier chapters, I've been living in a kind of emotional fog. Everything twirled slightly out of sync. Even my longtime personal relationship with God suffered.

Now, every now and again I sense a slight thaw. The pain subsides a bit. An hysterical crying binge does not follow every little whiff of Ron's aftershave. Will I freeze again? I expect so, but not for as long as the last time. With Christ at my side, I'll be able to handle it.

Dear friend, guard Clear Thinking and Common Sense with your life; don't for a minute lose sight of them.

They'll keep your soul alive and well, they'll keep you fit and attractive. You'll travel safely, you'll neither tire nor trip. You'll take afternoon naps without a worry, you'll enjoy a good night's sleep. No need to panic over alarms or surprises, or predictions that doomsday's just around the corner, Because God will be right there with you; he'll keep you safe and sound (Proverbs 3:21–26, MSG).

This week, I attended both a funeral and a 50th wedding anniversary. Not a great combination. Thankfully, I found myself surrounded by good friends and family at each occasion. I saved my worst reactions for the ride home alone. And there is nothing to do but just keep walking forward into the pain, because if I don't, God can't get a grasp on it to soothe it with His grace. Oh but for the grace of God, what would I ever do?

While Psalm 6 described my original misery to a tee, now it is only true some of the time.

Have mercy on me and be gracious to me, O Lord, for I am weak (faint and withered away); O Lord, heal me, for my bones are troubled. My [inner] self [as well as my body] is also exceedingly disturbed and troubled. But You, O Lord, how long [until You return and speak peace to me]? Return [to my relief], O Lord, deliver my life; save me for the sake of Your steadfast love and mercy…I am weary with my groaning; all night I soak my pillow with tears, I drench my couch with my weeping (Psalm 6:2-6).

Ten Months Now

Mondays are difficult. I notice the emptiness more on Mondays for some reason. My heart is especially heavy today. So instead of eating, I write. The TV blares behind me, but I don't really hear the show blaring in the background…until I hear the words to

THE PREGNANT PAUSE OF GRIEF

this song. "If tomorrow never comes, will she know how much I love her? Will she know how much I care…?"

And the grace of God pours over me again as I listen to the words of the song Ron chose for his funeral service. Of course, I cried. Then I wondered if I'd recovered in any way at all, until friend and fellow author Patricia Day sent her blogpost. Here is an excerpt.

> A close friend is dealing with the loss of her husband. She finds some days interminably long and difficult. However hard the day, she busies herself in a myriad of ways. She is an awesome role model and an inspiration. She is a writer and a public motivational speaker. She is actively involved in women's ministries at our church. She busies herself helping others, and then when she can—she finds time for herself. That is the harder part, because she is still trying to discover who or what she is now she is no longer a wife.
>
> To me, she is strong and positive and productive, yet she admits she sometimes closes the front door to her home and collapses in tears. Loneliness is a deep, dark place that is only lit from within the heart, as you manage to overcome the aloneness and take those brave new steps into a world that is waiting for you to live.
>
> My dear friend is doing all the right things but still has moments of despair. Nobody can understand the feelings of grief until they have experienced the loss of someone they loved (http://pepeprays.wordpress.com).

Almost One Year

According to something I read, the first anniversary of Ron's death will be particularly heart rending because I will realize that Ron is not coming back. Quite frankly, I figured that out on the day he died.

God has been faithful for the last 364 days. I doubt that He will change on day 365. I determine to thank Him for all the wonderful years Ron and I had together. I will thank God that Ron is free from any more pain and suffering. I'll mention the loving family, friends, neighbours, and even strangers, who cared for me in so many ways these last months.

The Dreaded Day
I can't believe it's a year already. I never knew the journey would be so hard or that I would feel so exposed. Perhaps other widows said something, but if they did, I don't recall it. I do however remember the hollow look in their eyes. That should have given me a hint.

We who have been loved and cherished find ourselves suddenly uncovered—that is, unprotected, exposed to the world—because our loved one is gone. Thank God for the One who is willing to take up that stance for us.

Fear not, for you shall not be ashamed; neither be confounded and depressed, for you shall not be put to shame. For you shall forget the shame of your youth, and you shall not [seriously] remember the reproach of your widowhood any more. For your Maker is your Husband—the Lord of hosts is His name—and the Holy One of Israel is your Redeemer; the God of the whole earth He is called. For the Lord has called you like a woman forsaken, grieved in spirit, and heartsore—even a wife [wooed and won] in youth, when she is [later] refused and scorned, says your God (Isaiah 54:4–6).

I had to write the newspaper notice weeks before. Now it stares me in the face, as if I could possibly have forgotten the day.

So, my dearest Ronald... We rejoice with you as you enjoy heaven, even though our hearts continue to miss you. We strive to be the family you cared so well for, because you were always the beloved Husband, Dad and Afi we needed. You need not worry about us. God is covering for you... Love from Brenda and family.

INTO THE SECOND YEAR

Listen! Whatever you are going through right now, you can survive it. At some point you will even begin to thrive, because God is enough. It is just over a year since my heart broke, and little by little, it heals. The scars remain, but if I don't pick at them too much I can get through the day. "*But You, O Lord, are a shield for me, my glory, and the lifter of my head*" (Psalm 3:3).

I started a "thank you" page listing those who made my journey a bit easier, but I ran out of room. You know who you are. You listened, and you let me cry. You brought meals and invited me to events. You worried about my finances and my spiritual health. You prayed for me and with me. You read books on grief so you could relate. You hugged me and sent encouragement by phone, letter, email, and text.

I offer a special thank you to those who've already walked this road of grief. You know what it feels like to be alone and unprotected. You understand about learning new skills and taking on added responsibility. You too sometimes feel that you no longer belong anywhere. Most of all, you set the bar for recovery.

To sum it all up, God is sufficient, but He works through people. Thank you, one and all. Your presence in my life made this grief journey bearable.

> *All praise to the God and Father of our Master, Jesus the Messiah! Father of all mercy! God of all healing counsel! He comes alongside us when we go through hard times, and before you know it, he brings us alongside someone else who is going through hard times so that we can be there for that person just as God was there for us. We have plenty of hard times that come from following the Messiah, but no more so than the good times of his healing comfort—we get a full measure of that, too* (2 Corinthians 1:3-5, MSG).

FIFTEEN MONTHS LATER

Some question why I still cry. They only see the random teardrops that take effect without my permission. I wonder what they would say about the private ones. I do not apologize for missing the love of my life. Grief is the final gift for loving deeply.

I can't be with Ron, but I continue to follow the advice God gave me that scary day so long ago. "*I call heaven and earth to witness this day against you that I have set before you life and death, the blessings and the curses; therefore choose life, that you and your descendants may live*" (Deuteronomy 30:19).

Some married couples seem to thrive on bickering, insulting, and backbiting one another. I want to scream at them, "Some day you will regret this!"

I watch others who love like Ron and I did. I want to remind them to nourish and care for one another even more. Some day, they will wonder why they didn't pour even more life into their relationship.

As I see it, I need not be ashamed of loving so much that my grief never totally disappears. I am not weak because I still cry. I am not a failure because I still love.

Books surface from the authors' personal need to tell their story. Some people listen, but even the best of friends get weary of the same thing over and over. "*It was good of you to share in my troubles*" (Philippians 4:14, NIV).

Thank you, or as Ron would say, "Thank you muchly" for sharing this journey with me. May this book help you, in some small way, toward your own healing.

Sincerely,
Brenda J. Wood

THE END

Epilogue

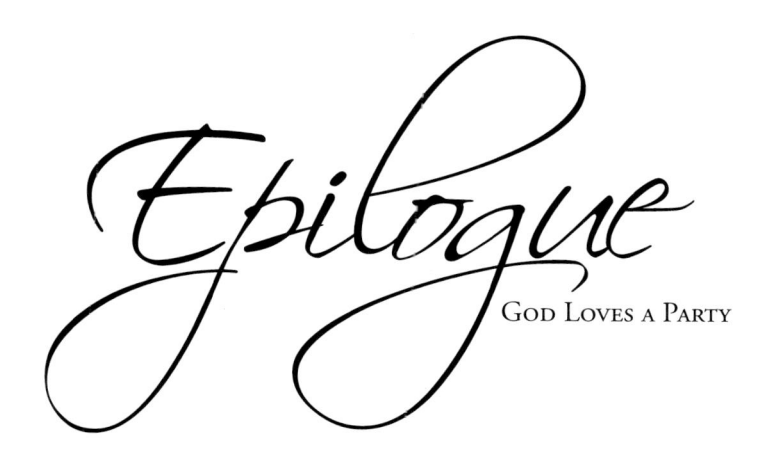

God Loves a Party

Months ago, still in the depths of grief, I was asked to do a speaking event on March 2, 2013. Because of the circumstances, I recognized God's hand in it and promptly agreed to go. That's why I'm travelling to a speaking engagement on our fiftieth wedding anniversary.

Ron and I always wanted to have a big celebration on our fiftieth. Today I face it alone. Yet not alone, because God is throwing me a fiftieth wedding anniversary party! The guest list even includes relatives and friends who just happen go to this particular church.

I am excited, fearful, anxious, sad, depressed, happy and adventurous all at the same time as I travel several hours through a Canadian winter, to the biggest party of my life.

"If you'll hold on to me for dear life," says God, "I'll get you out of any trouble. I'll give you the best of care if you'll only get to know and trust me. Call me and I'll answer, be at your side in bad times; I'll rescue you, then throw you a party. I'll give you a long life, give you a long drink of salvation!" (Psalm 91:13-15, MSG)

I don't know why I'm so surprised. After all, God delights in giving us the desires of our heart! (Psalm 37:4)